LAPAROSCOPIC SURGERY

Edited by **Arshad M. Malik**

Laparoscopic Surgery
http://dx.doi.org/10.5772/62675
Edited by Arshad M. Malik

Contributors

Francisco M. Sánchez-Margallo, Juan A. Sánchez Margallo, Javier Hermoso De Mendoza, David Zimmerman, Stefan Clermonts, Laurents Stassen, Thomas Lango, Erlend Hofstad, Ronald Mårvik, Chih-Kun Huang, Prasad Madhusudan Bhukebag, Sir Emmanuel Astudillo, Khan Wei Chan, Alessandro M. Paganini, Andrea Balla, Silvia Quaresima, Ardit Seitaj, Andrea Isidori, Franco Iafrate, Arshad M Malik

Published by InTech
Janeza Trdine 9, 51000 Rijeka, Croatia

Publishing Process Manager Martina Usljebrka
Technical Editor SPi Global
Cover InTech Design team

First published February, 2017
Printed in Croatia
Legal deposit, Croatia: National and University Library in Zagreb

Additional hard copies can be obtained from orders@intechopen.com

Laparoscopic Surgery, Edited by Arshad M. Malik
p. cm.
Print ISBN 978-953-51-2963-9
Online ISBN 978-953-51-2964-6

For EU product safety concerns:
IN TECH d.o.o., Prolaz Marije Krucifikse Kozulić 3, 51000 Rijeka, Croatia,
info@intechopen.com or visit our website at intechopen.com.

Meet the editor

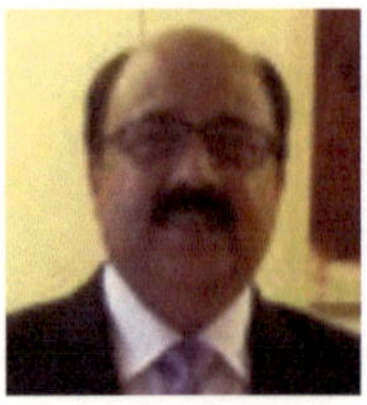

Dr. Arshad M. Malik is an associate professor of Surgery at the College of Medicine, Department of Surgery, Qassim University, Saudi Arabia. He developed special interest in laparoscopic surgery and then got training in India and Singapore, to name a few. Presently he is an assistant editor of the *International Journal of Health Sciences* which is an official journal of Qassim University. He is a reviewer of the *British Journal of Medical Practitioners* as well as many other international journals. He is the author of 46 national and international scientific papers which are well appreciated in the health community. He is the editor of one book on *Advances in Laparoscopic Surgery* wherein he has contributed one chapter on the laparoscopic appendectomy. His chapter on "The Recent Trends in the Management of Appendicular Mass" has attracted a massive readership and has been downloaded for 17,000 times all over the world. He has been presenting his work on the floor of many well-established and renowned surgical and laparoscopic societies like ELSA, SLS, APHS, WCES, IAGES, EAES, EHS, and AHS in India, Italy, Spain, New York, Los Angeles, Yokohama, Belgium, Indonesia, Singapore, Vietnam, etc., to name a few. His work has been appreciated and well taken by the experts in this field.

Contents

Preface

The present era has seen a revolution in the field of surgery where there has been a dramatic shift from the traditional open surgery to minimal access surgery. This change is not an overnight phenomenon but a result of vision, hard work, and dedication of many individuals over the past few decades. The early pioneers planted the seeds which, with a continuum of the same struggle by the present experts in this field, have expanded to and have become a huge tree of the modern present-day laparoscopy with many branches emerging every day.

We can still find patients, operated before the dawn of laparoscopic era, carrying big incisions on the operative sites. At the outset, most of the surgeons who were trained for open surgery were very reluctant and did not show eagerness to learn this technique. Soon it was realized that the laparoscopic surgery will not gain widespread acceptance unless the training of this technique is offered to surgeons all over the world. At that time, there was a dearth of properly trained medical and paramedical personnel, and there were very few properly qualified and trained surgeons who took this as a challenge to bring a phenomenal change to improve the outlook of surgical patients. It did not take very long when we saw surgeons developing an unfailing interest in learning and practicing this technique. I remember very clearly when I started the minimal access surgery, there were hardly few operations performed like cholecystectomy, appendectomy, etc. On the contrary, there was a long list of contraindications to laparoscopic surgery. This is attributed to lack of well-trained manpower as well as lack of properly trained paramedical staff and lack of recognized training programs and also the learning curve of this technique. Now as evident from studies from all over the world, there seems to be virtually no contraindications to the laparoscopic procedures, and almost every procedure is being performed through this technique.

Initially, the procedure gained popularity as it was associated with less pain, short hospital stay, and rapid recovery. The initial basic principles of the basic procedures were well taken and got established very early and at a very fast pace. Later on, all the energy was focused on the various advance procedures which were not performed as commonly as the basic laparoscopic procedures like cholecystectomy and appendectomy. Later on, the cosmetic gain of this technique attracted a worldwide popularity and people started working on this aspect. This led to the emergence of various advancements in this technique to make it more and more sophisticated in terms of cosmetic results and improvement in the operating techniques. Now people are more in the practice of scarless surgery, whereby patients have no obvious scar on the body. This target is being achieved by SILS, natural orifice transluminal endoscopic surgery (NOTES), etc. which is now gaining worldwide popularity. Robotic sur-

gery is a further advancement in this field gaining global acceptance, and a large number of centers are performing robotic surgery as a routine.

This book is just a step forward for the readers to learn further the diagnostic and therapeutic value of this novel technique. I hope that it will be a great help for the junior laparoscopic surgeons as well as it will attract attention of those who are routinely performing the laparoscopic surgery.

Any positive criticisms/suggestions are more than welcome.

Dr. Arshad M. Malik
Associate Professor, Surgery
College of Medicine
Qassim University
Saudi Arabia

Chapter 1

The Evolution of Minimally Invasive Techniques in Restoration of Colonic Continuity

Stefan H.E.M. Clermonts, Laurents P.S. Stassen and David D.E. Zimmerman

Additional information is available at the end of the chapter

http://dx.doi.org/10.5772/66720

Abstract

Restoration of bowel continuity after Hartmann's procedure is considered technically challenging and is associated with high morbidity and mortality. This is the main reason why restoration of intestinal continuity is often not attempted. Over the past decade, considerable international experience has gained on this topic with new minimally invasive techniques being developed. This review details the evolution of minimally invasive techniques in restoration of colonic continuity after Hartmann's procedure. A comprehensive search of PubMed and Embase was done. Different restoration modalities were included. Eight studies, from six different countries, in which multiport laparoscopic restoration of continuity was compared to conventional open restoration of bowel continuity, were included. In the total of 254 patients, continuity was restored laparoscopically compared with 255 patients in which continuity was performed in open fashion. Restoration of bowel continuity via trephine access was also reported; three studies including 37 patients were included in this review. Single-port restoration of bowel continuity after Hartmann's procedure is a natural evolution of multiport laparoscopy and trephine access. Six studies reporting on single-port reversal of Hartmann's procedure were included with a total of 75 patients. Single-port access in combination with a transanal approach has also been reported; however, data are extremely limited as there is only one study in the published literature. Success of restoration of bowel continuity with less morbidity and mortality has been demonstrated throughout the evolution of the different surgical techniques. In this review advantages of different approaches for restoration of bowel continuity after Hartmann's procedure are discussed. Furthermore, surgical techniques are described, pictorial guides are added for some techniques, and flowcharts are given for easy use during clinical decision-making.

Keywords: Hartmann's procedure, restoration, intestinal continuity, surgical techniques, laparoscopic, minimal invasive, single-port laparoscopy

1. Introduction

In this chapter we would like to focus on the restoration of intestinal continuity after Hartmann's procedure in general and highlight emerging minimally invasive techniques in specific.

Historically, restoration of bowel continuity after Hartmann's procedure has been considered technically challenging and is associated with high morbidity and mortality rates even despite modern surgical techniques. This is the main reason why restoration of intestinal continuity is often not attempted. Intraoperative difficulties during laparotomy or multi-port laparoscopy are mainly caused by the formation of adhesions at the laparotomy site and lower part of the abdomen after active inflammation and/or infection and previous surgery.

The use of the former colostomy site as access to the abdominal cavity has gained some popularity recently. Placing a single-port access system in the former colostomy site combines the potential benefits of minimally invasive surgery (shorter postoperative recovery time, minimal postoperative hospital stay, and lower morbidity rates) with the advantages of Hartmann's reversal through the colostomy site (the absence of new incisions and decreased necessity of midline adhesiolysis).

2. Hartmann's procedure: historical perspective

Henri Albert Hartmann was born on June 16, 1860. Hartmann finished his medical school at the University of Paris on December 19, 1881.

Hartmann starts his internship with Felix Terrier at Hôpital Bichat, who was considered to be one of the most authoritative surgeons at that time [1]. After finishing his surgical training in 1887, Hartmann was appointed as an assistant professor in 1895 and in 1909 as a professor and chairman of the Department of Surgery in 1892. In 1914, Hartman became the chief of Surgery at l'Hôtel-Dieu hospital in Paris (**Figure 1**) [2]. During his lengthy and extraordinary career, Hartmann meticulously recorded each operation he performed. Upon his retirement he had documented around 30,000 cases [3].

Hartmann's procedure was first described in 1921 [4, 5]. In his first patients with obstructive carcinoma of the sigmoid, he performed a proximal colostomy and then a sigmoid resection with closure of the rectal stump via an abdominal approach. He developed this technique in response to high mortality rates in his patients who underwent an abdominoperineal resection, as first described by Miles in 1908 [1]. In 1931 Hartmann described the procedure in detail in his book *Chirurgie du Rectum* (**Figure 2**).

Although Hartmann developed his technique mainly for rectal cancer, in present times, Hartmann's procedure is often the preferred procedure for severe diverticulitis of the sigmoid. Despite Hartmann never intended restoration of bowel continuity, recent publications showed that a direct reconstruction is feasible in selected patients [6].

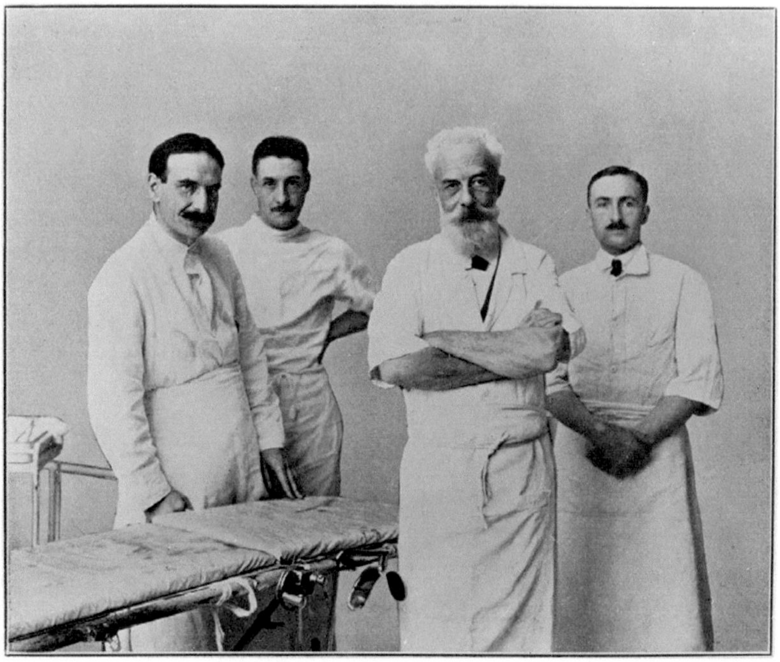

Figure 1. Henri Hartmann (second from the right) and his three assistants, Drs. Bergeret, Gouverneur, and Huet, at the Hotel-Dieu, Paris. Source image: http://wellcomeimages.org.

2.1. Reversal of Hartmann's procedure

Hartmann never attempted to reanastomose the bowel in his patients. He believed this would result in unnecessarily high morbidity and mortality [3].

Restoring intestinal continuity after Hartmann's operation is a difficult operation that is associated with a high morbidity rate, with anastomotic leakage rates ranging from 4% to 16% and an operative mortality reported as high as 10% [7–10].

The high incidence of morbidity and mortality is the main reasons why surgeons are reluctant to restore intestinal continuity in approximately 40% of the patients undergoing Hartmann's procedure [10, 11].

2.2. Indications and contraindications

The primary indication for reversal of Hartmann's procedure is curing people of the discomforts that are caused by the end colostomy. Patients with stomas face many physical and psychological challenges, including leakage, skin rashes, lifestyle alterations, and sexual dysfunction [12, 13].

Literature defines no contraindications for reversal of Hartmann's procedure. However, a review of the literature covering restoration after Hartmann's procedure shows that advanced age, ASA grade 3, or higher and fecal peritonitis at the time of Hartmann's procedure are

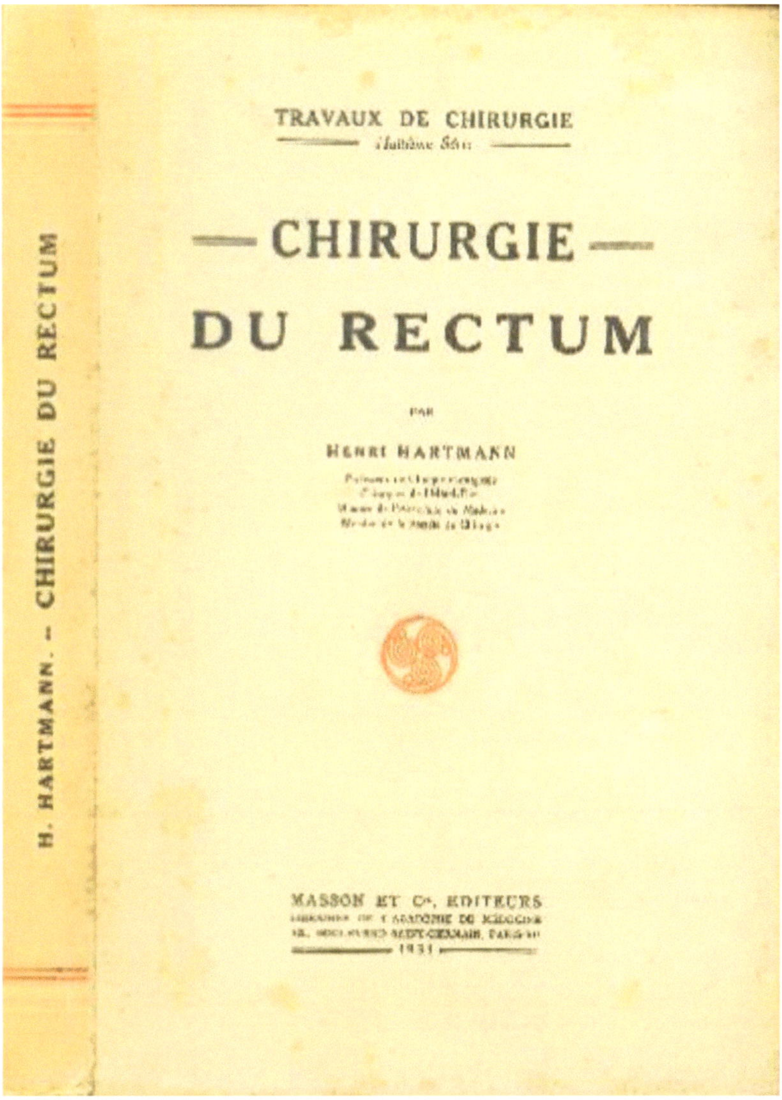

Figure 2. Cover of the book *Chirurgie du rectum* by Henri Hartmann. Published 1931. Source image: http://archive.org.

often considered relevant contraindications. Roque-Castellano and colleagues analyzed factors related to the decision of restoring intestinal continuity. They found that female sex and neoplastic disorders are relative contraindications for restoration of intestinal continuity [14]. Furthermore, we believe there must be some reluctance to perform conventional restoration of bowel continuity by laparotomy in patients with an incisional hernia. The reason for this statement is the need for repair of the incisional hernia and the restoration of the bowel continuity at the same time. This reluctance is following the dictum that abdominal wall prostheses must be avoided during contaminated operations [15]. The authors advocate

the use of single-port laparoscopic reversal of Hartmann's procedure in case of an incisional hernia. With this modality the midline can be left unchanged rendering concomitant repair of the incisional hernia unnecessary. The single-port laparoscopic technique will be discussed in detail in Section 5.1.

2.3. Preoperative workup

Prior to the restoration of the intestinal continuity, routine evaluation of the rectal stump and descending colon is often performed in order to detect stump leakage, cavity formation, or strictures and establish the length of the rectal stump. The integrity and patency of the rectal stump are evaluated by physical examination, flexible endoscopy and/or radiographically by contrast proctography CT scan. Despite these routine practices, little data exist to support this in case of restoration of bowel continuity after Hartmann's procedure. Data do exist on the routine use of contrast enema prior to the closure of a defunctioning ileostomy in patients with low pelvic anastomosis is inconsistent when its sole purpose is detecting leaks or cavity formation [16–18]. These studies show that strictures or narrowing of the bowel lumen is seldom detected. In cases where strictures are detected, dilatation is performed without the need for cancelation the reversal of the – ostomy. When extrapolating these findings, it is questionable whether routine contrast studies are necessary in the case of Hartmann's reversal. Moreover, usually patients who develop an anastomotic leak of the rectal stump present with clinical symptoms long before restoration of the bowel continuity is scheduled. However, in patients where initial Hartmann's procedure was acutely performed for neoplastic disorders, direct visualization of the rectal stump and remaining colon is mandatory to exclude recurrence of the malignancy or other neoplastic lesions. Based on these limited data, the authors advocate performing flexible rectoscopy to ensure viability of the rectal stump and the absence of remaining diverticular disease or local recurrence in case of prior malignancy. Data on routinely performing X-ray or contrast enema is limited to expert opinions and therefore not mandatory. Authors' recommendations are summarized in the algorithm in **Figure 3**.

2.4. Timing of surgery

There is limited data available concerning the optimal timing of restoration of continuity. Most surgeons will postpone surgery for at least 6 months after the initial operation, obviously depending on the current health and recuperation of the patient. It has been suggested by Keck and coworkers that a waiting period of 15 weeks may be beneficial [19]. It is however noteworthy that reversing Hartmann's procedure after a shorter period did not influence morbidity or mortality, but did seem to lengthen the duration of hospitalisation and increase the perceived operative difficulty (and thus the risk). Other authors have also suggested there is no indication to delay closure for longer than 16 weeks [20]. Based on these limited data, the authors advocate a minimal waiting period of 4 months between the initial operation and restoration of continuity in order to maximize the possibility of minimally invasive techniques for restoring continuity.

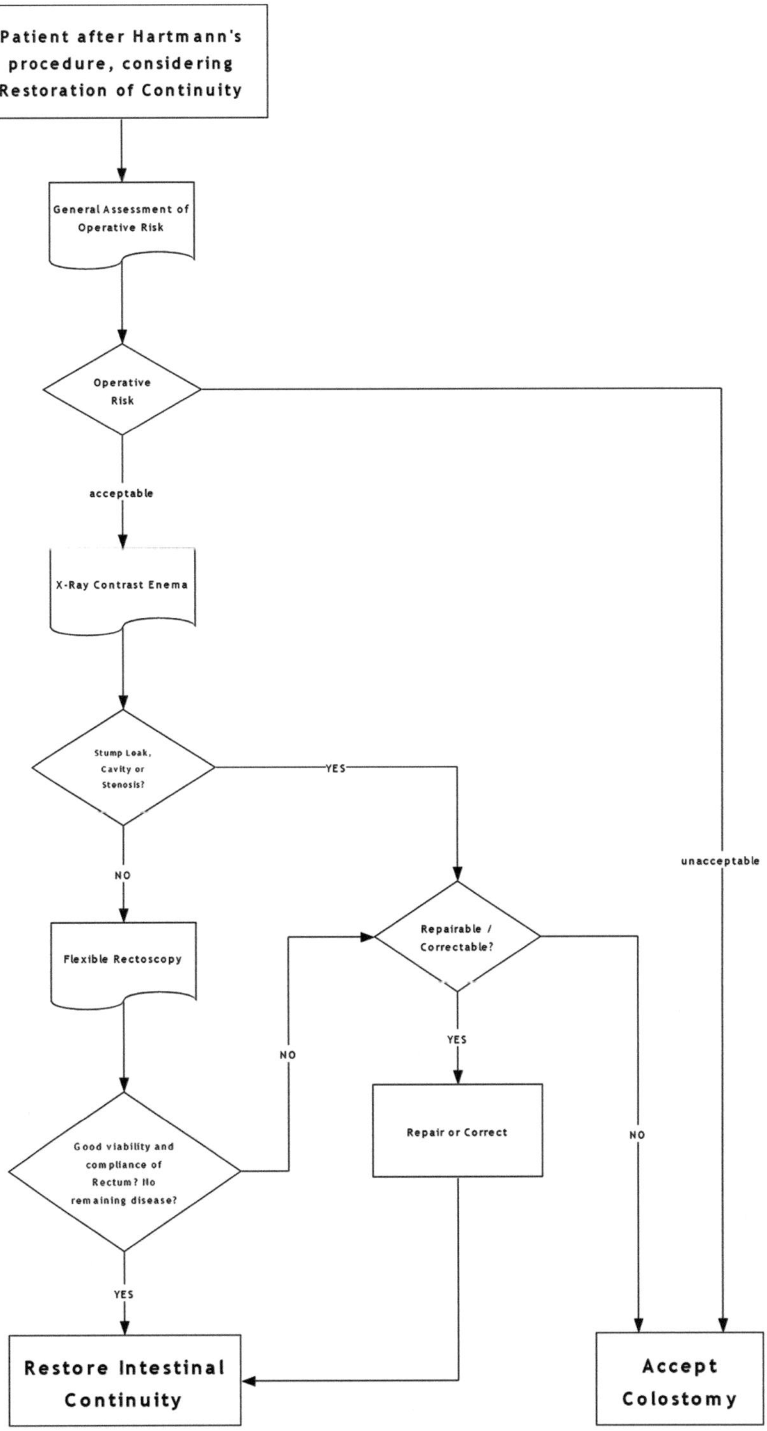

Figure 3. Algorithm advocated to be used during decision-making and the preoperative workup for restoration of bowel continuity after Hartmann's procedure.

http://dx.doi.org/10.5772/66720

3. Surgical techniques for restoration of intestinal continuity after Hartmann's procedure

Reestablishing bowel continuity after Hartmann's procedure is considered a major surgical procedure that is accompanied by considerable morbidity and mortality. Multiport laparoscopy was the first technique in a sequence of attempts to reduce the high morbidity and mortality that is associated with this procedure.

3.1. Multiport laparoscopic reversal of Hartmann's procedure

The patient is placed in a supine position. Next, there are two different ways to continue the procedure. In one option the procedure is initiated with mobilization of the stoma to the level of the abdominal wall and then freeing the ostomy from the fascia. The alternative procedure starts by insertion of a 10 mm camera trocar and a working trocar when needed (**Figure 4**), establishing the pneumoperitoneum, and perform a prior inspection for factors that could potentially cause abortion later on in the procedure. We advocate starting the procedure in the latter fashion, since this technique facilitates early decision-making by the surgeon on continuing or aborting the procedure when a potential unsuccessful bowel restoration is anticipated. Consequently, there is no need for refashioning of the end colostomy.

In both techniques the next step is transecting the colon using a linear stapler to remove the end of the colostomy and securing the anvil of a circular stapler is secured with a purse-string suture, in the proximal colon. The descending colon is then returned into the abdominal cavity. Any adhesions in the abdominal cavity are freed to enable insertion of the other ports. The colostomy site is closed using a wound protector/retractor device with a laparoscopic cap so that it can function as an additional working port. The pneumoperitoneum is then established. Additional 5 mm working trocars are placed in the right upper quadrant and right iliac fossa. Extensive dissection of adhesions from the anterior abdominal wall in the midline is mandatory with this multi-port technique in order to cross the midline (**Figure 4**).

The small bowel is mobilized from the left iliac fossa and out of the pelvis. The proximal descending colon would have been mobilized to a varying extent at the initial Hartmann's procedure, and this will need to be redone, including the splenic flexure. A rectal probe or circular stapler sizer is used to identify the rectal stump. In order to perform an end-to-end anastomosis, further mobilization and adhesiolysis of the rectal stump are sometimes necessary. Alternatively, if mobilization is difficult and the anterior rectal wall can clearly be identified and adequate length of the descending colon is available to allow a tension-free anastomosis, an side-to-side anastomosis can be performed. A circular stapler is introduced into the rectum to fashion the anastomosis. The stapler is deployed and the donuts are checked. Next, we advocate performing an additional leak test as this is associated with reduced rates of postoperative adverse events in literature [21]. The pneumoperitoneum is released, and the trocars are removed under direct visualization. The fascia is then closed in apertures equal to or larger than 10 mm.

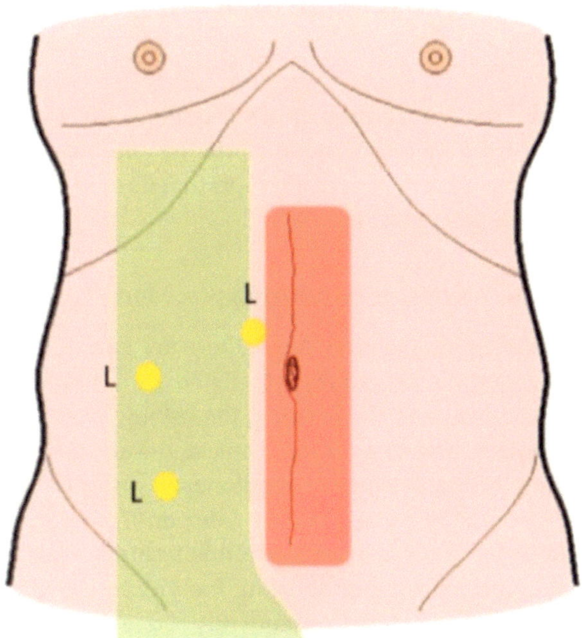

Figure 4. Port positions for multiport laparoscopic Hartmann's reversal. L = laparoscopic trocar position. *Red-shaded area*: area of maximal adhesion formation after previous laparotomy. *Green-shaded area*: area of range of action that is relatively free of adhesions. Note that in this technique the midline has to be crossed.

3.2. The open technique compared to multiport laparoscopic restoration technique: an appraisal of the literature

In recent literature a limited amount of studies compared an open approach with the multiport laparoscopic technique [22–31]. In **Table 1** a summary of studies on multiport laparoscopic versus conventional Hartmann's reversal is presented.

As expected, for the minimal invasive technique, the total length of hospital stay was shorter with 6.9 days when compared to the open approach that shows a mean of 10.4 days. Furthermore, for patients in whom bowel continuity was restored laparoscopically, overall morbidity rates seemed lower when compared to patients who were treated conventionally. In the laparoscopic group, mean morbidity rates were 12% versus 20% in the open group. The main and foremost complications after bowel restoration for both modalities are summarized in **Table 2**.

In the reviewed literature, mortality seems comparable for both techniques, with a mean mortality of 0.9% in the laparoscopic group and 1.2% in the conventional group. No statistically significant differences were found for mean total operation time, 150 minutes for the laparoscopic technique and 172 minutes for conventional procedures. A possible explanation for the relative long operation duration for both techniques is the extensive adhesiolysis that is required. 80 percent of the conversions from laparoscopy to the conventional technique arises for this reason [33], resulting in an average conversion rate of 12 percent. In the opinion of the authors, there is no place for primary open restoration of continuity after Hartmann's

http://dx.doi.org/10.5772/66720

Study	Country	Year of publication	Procedure	Number of patients	Morbidity (%)	Mortality (%	Operation time (mean min)	Hospital stay (days)	Control group (number of patients)	Morbidity (%)	Mortality (%)	Operation time (mean min)	Hospital stay (days)
Rosen et al. [24]	USA	2005	Laparoscopic	20	3 (14)	0 (0)	158	4.2	No				NS
Faure et al. [25]	FR	2007	Laparoscopic	14	2(14.2)	0 (0)	143	9.5	Conventional (20)	6 (30)	0 (0)	180	11
Haughn et al. [26]	USA	2008	Laparoscopic	61	8 (13)	0 (0)	154	NS	Conventional (61)	11 (18)	0(0)	210	NS
Vermeulen et al. [27]	NL	2008	Laparoscopic	3	(15.8)*	(5)*	NS	NS	Conventional(48)	(15.8)*	(5)*	NS	NS
Mazeh et al. [28]	IL	2009	Laparoscopic	82	15 (17.6)	0 (0)	193	6.5	Conventional (41)	15 (36.5)	0 (0)	209	8.1
Di Carlo et al. [29]	IT	2010	Laparoscopic	3	0 (0)	0 (0)	95.6	NS	Conventional (3)	0 (0)	0 (0)	136.6	NS
De'angelis et al. [30]	FR	2013	Laparoscopic	28	3 (10.7)	0 (0)	171.1	6.7	Conventional (18)	6 (33.6)	0 (0)	235.8	11.2
Yang et al. [31]	AU	2014	Laparoscopic	43	6 (14)	0 (0)	276.4	6.7	Conventional (64)	20 (31)	0 (0)	242	10.8

AU, Australia; FR, France; IT, Italy; IL, Israel; NL, the Netherlands; USA, United States of America; NS, not stated.In the study by Vermeulen et al. [32]. Subdivision is made for laparoscopic or conventional reversal; therefore, only overall morbidity and mortality are given for this study.

Table 1. Summary of current literature that compares multiport laparoscopic Hartmann's reversal versus the conventional open technique.

	Type of intestinal continuity restoration	
	Multiport laparoscopy	Laparotomy
Hemorrhage	1.7	3
Wound infection	10.6	14
Anastomotic leakage	1.2	5
Reoperation	4	7
Cardiopulmonary	3.6	7

Values are derived from the literature. Values are in mean percentages.

Table 2. Morbidity rates depicted for multiport laparoscopic reversal of Hartmann's procedure compared with conventional reversal.

procedure, due to unnecessary morbidity, mortality, and trauma to the abdominal wall. We advocate selection of a minimally invasive procedure.

4. Trephine access: using the former colostomy site as access point

Although laparoscopic restoration of the intestinal continuity has many advantages, in laparoscopic reversal of Hartmann's procedure, an extended adhesiolysis in the midline and pelvis is still needed. This adhesiolysis may increase postoperative paralytic ileus and the risk of inadvertent bowel lacerations.

The use of the colostomy site as an even less invasive method for access to the abdominal cavity and restoration of the intestinal continuity was first described by Vermeulen and colleagues in 2008 [32]. In this technique manual access is gained through the stoma site in combination with a blindly performed adhesiolysis without laparoscopic assistance (**Figure 5**). This procedure was called the SIR method "stoma incision reversal" procedure.

4.1. SIR procedure: surgical technique

The patient is positioned in the lithotomy. The stoma is released, taking a small amount of surrounding skin with it. Then the colostomy is closed provisionally with a running suture. The length of the incision at the stomal site must be large enough to fit the surgeon's hand. The descending colon stump is brought outside the abdomen; visible adhesions connected to the left colon are sharply dissected. Further adhesiolysis of the left colon is performed manually between the thumb and index finger in order to create enough length for the descending colon to reach the pelvic cavity. If enough bowel length is created. The anvil of a circular stapler is placed intraluminal. The stump is closed using a linear stapler. The tip of the stapler anvil is brought through the colon the staple line and tied by a purse-string suture. The descending colon with the anvil is returned intra-abdominally. For the next step, the surgeon's right hand is placed intra-abdominally through the former colostomy side. The left hand is used to transanally introduce a rigid sizer to identify and manipulate the rectal stump. Adhesions between the rectal stump and adjacent small bowels are loosened manually and blindly with the surgeon's right hand. Consecutively, the circular stapler is introduced into

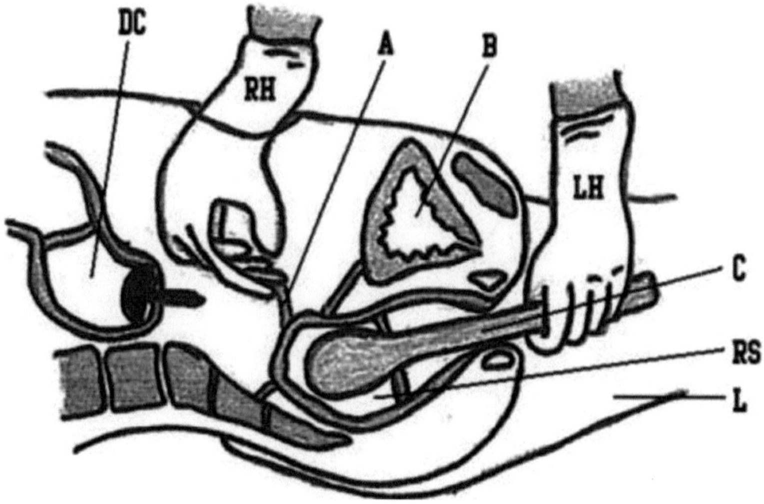

Figure 5. Manual lysis of adhesions at the tip of the rectal stump, which was identified using a rigid club. Previously, the anvil of a circular stapler was placed intraluminal of the descending colon. DC, descending colon with anvil; RH, right hand; A, adhesions; B, bladder; LH, left hand; C, rigid club; RS, rectal stump; L, left leg. Source: Ref. [34].

the rectal stump. The pin of the circular stapler is passed through the rectal wall, and the anvil is attached. Before firing the circular stapler, the proximal bowel segment is manually checked for rotation and interposition. After firing the stapler, the integrity of the doughnuts of the anastomosis is inspected, and a leak test is performed. The fascia is closed with a PDS suture, and the skin as deemed appropriate.

4.2. Appraisal of the literature

A review of the literature shows three studies [32, 34–36] on the SIR technique. **Table 3** summarizes the results. Vermeulen and colleagues described the first pilot study in 2010. They attempted the procedure in 13 consecutive patients with a median age of 56 years (range 35–81 years). Indications for initial surgery were iatrogenic bowel perforation ($n = 3$), intestinal bowel obstruction due to complicated diverticulitis ($n = 3$), and diverticulitis ($n = 7$). Median delay of reversal was 7 months.

Of the 13 patients assigned for reversal of Hartmann's procedure through the stomal site, two patients needed direct conversion to laparotomy due to firm adhesions. Of the 11 patients in which the procedure was accomplished through the stoma site, mean operation time was 81 min (range 58–109 min) with a mean hospital stay of 4.2 days. No anastomotic leaks occurred. In 2010 Vermeulen and colleagues published the results of their "stoma incision reversal" procedure in 22 patients and compare the results with matched cases in which restoration of the intestinal continuity was performed by laparotomy. In the "SIR" group, five procedures were converted to laparotomy due to firm adhesions ($n = 2$), doubt about the quality of the doughnuts ($n = 2$), or iatrogenic small bowel lacerations ($n = 1$).

In this study the mean operation time was significantly shorter when performing the SIR procedure (75 min (58–208)) compared to the open group (141 min (85–276)) ($p < 0.001$). Patients

Study	Country	Year of publication	Number of patients	Procedure	Control group (number of patients)	Morbidity (%)	Mortality (%)	Operation time (mean min)	Hospital stay (days)
Vermeulen et al. [32]	NL	2008	13	Trephine access	No (0)	0 (0)	0 (0)	81	4.2
Vermeulen et al. [34]	NL	2010	16	Trephine access	Yes (32)	4 (25)	0 (0)	75	4
Aydin et al. [35]	TR	2011	8	Trephine access	No (0)	0 (0)	0	65	5.5

NL, the Netherlands; TR, Turkey.

Table 3. Summary of "trephine access" technique reversal of Hartmann's procedure in the current literature.

	Type of intestinal continuity restoration	
	"SIR"	Laparotomy
Total complications	4	16
Anastomotic leakage	1	2
Ileus	0	1
Wound infections	1	5
Urine retention	1	0
Incisional hernia	1	8
Mortality	0	1
Vermeulen et al. 2010 [35].		

Table 4. Postoperative complications after restoration of bowel continuity depicted for the "SIR" procedure (trephine access) and conventional technique.

who underwent the SIR procedure had a shorter postoperative hospital stay (SIR group range 2-7 days) ($p < 0.001$). The total postoperative number of complications was not significantly different between both procedures. Twenty-five percent for the SIR patients versus 50% of the patients that were treated by the conventional technique. Postoperative complications after bowel continuity restoration are depicted in **Table 4**.

In 2011 Aydin and colleagues perform the aforementioned technique in eight patients. Indications for the initial Hartmann's procedure were sigmoid volvulus ($n = 4$), obstructive sigmoid cancer ($n = 2$), rectal trauma ($n = 2$), and Fournier's gangrene ($n = 1$). The mean duration between the primary procedure and reversal of the Hartmann's procedure was 5 months (range 2–8 months). All patients included had a body mass index of less than 30 km/m^2 and a rectal stump of at least 5 cm. In two patients the incision was extended from the stoma site for better visualization of the rectal stump in one patient and due to injury of the intestine in one patient. Mean duration of the operation was 65 min (range 45–80 min). No postoperative complications were observed. Patients were discharged after a mean of 5.5 days (range 4–9 days). Aydin and coworkers note that this technique should ideally be used in non-obese patients with long rectal stumps of sufficient length.

The SIR technique originated in the Netherlands and met criticism due to the blind nature of the dissection phase of the procedure. Regarding the risk of blind dissection as well as the availability of improved access platforms that enable adequate vision and control, the authors do not advocate the use of the SIR technique in present times.

5. Single-port restoration of the intestinal continuity through the stoma trephine site

Single-port restoration of intestinal continuity with access through the formal site of the colostomy is a relatively new technique. The main goal for the development of this method is

introducing a minimally invasive technique that further reduces the morbidity and mortality of a procedure that is technically demanding and complex.

5.1. Surgical technique

The patient is placed in lithotomy position. Primarily, the colostomy is mobilized and freed from the fascia (**Figure 6**). The mobilized descending colon is then pulled out of the abdomen and exposed (**Figure 7**). Next, the colon is transected using a linear stapler to remove the end colostomy, and the anvil of a circular stapler is secured with a purse-string suture, in the proximal colon. Either a terminal or lateral position can be chosen (**Figure 8**). The descending colon is returned into the abdominal cavity. Any adhesions close to the wound in the abdominal cavity on direct view are freed. The single-port access platform is then placed in the fascial defect at the colostomy site, and the pneumoperitoneum is then established (**Figure 9**). A rigid 30-degree laparoscope is introduced and a diagnostic laparoscopy is performed. Subsequently, the patient

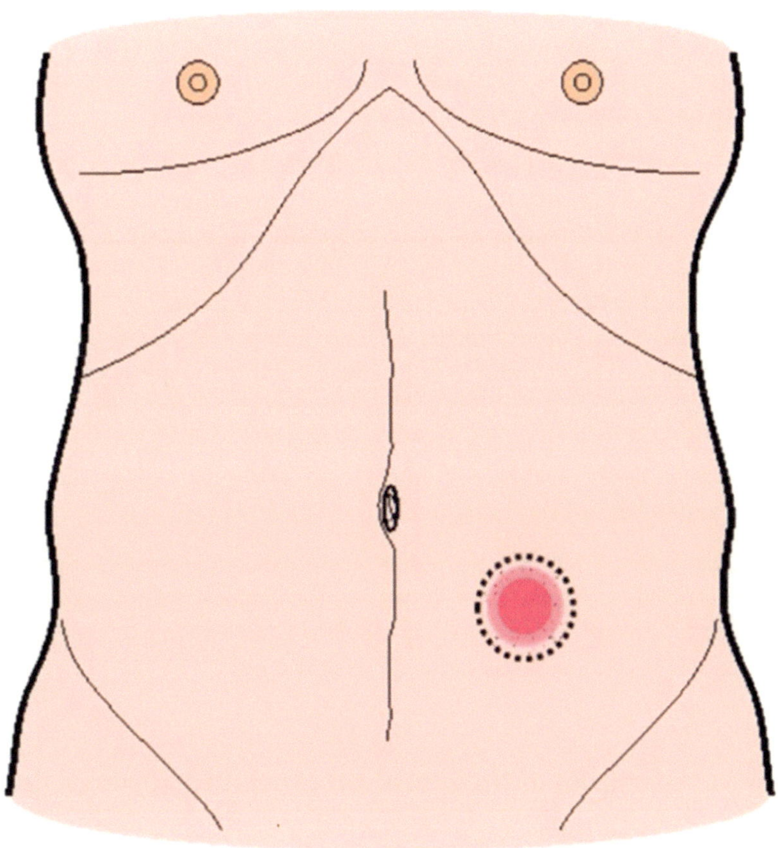

Figure 6. Release of the colostomy.

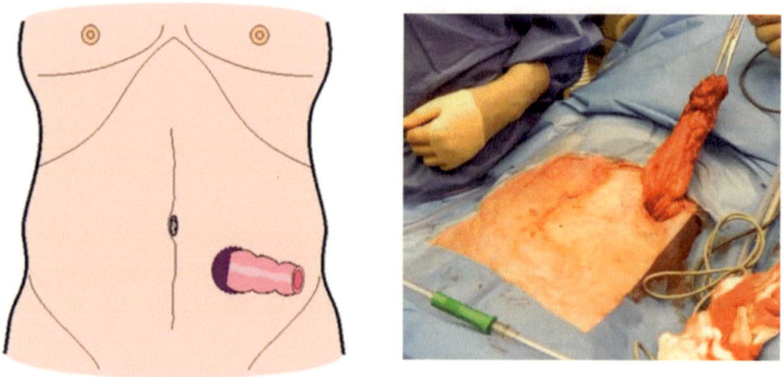

Figure 7. Mobilization of the descending colon with sufficient length.

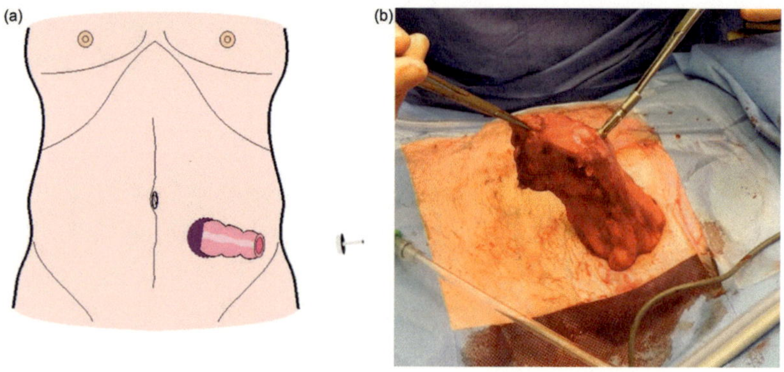

Figure 8. Insertion of the anvil of the circular stapler. Left picture shows a terminal position. Right picture shows a lateral positioning of the anvil for side-to-end configuration.

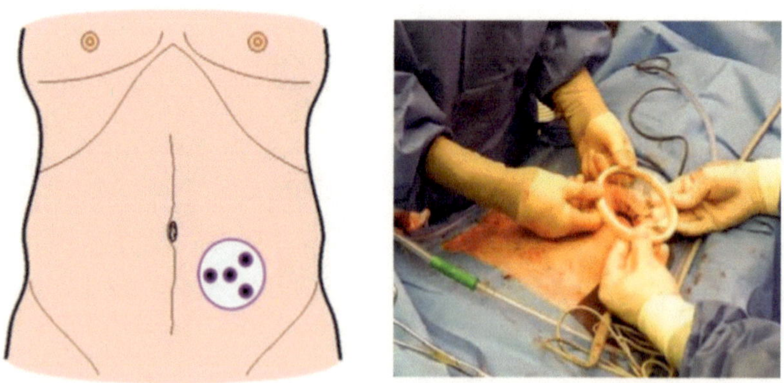

Figure 9. Placement of the single-port access device in the fascia defect at the formal stoma site. Right picture shows the placement of the flexible wound protector.

is positioned in anti-Trendelenburg position making the small pelvis visible. Adhesiolysis is performed using two 5 mm working trocars.

Dissection of adhesions and scar tissue surrounding the rectal stump is performed extensively, by either sharp dissection with laparoscopic scissors or ultrasonic dissection devices, until the rectal stump is as bare as possible (**Figure 10**). Adhesions formed at the previous midline incision can be left unchanged at this stage, reducing the risk of iatrogenic bowel perforation and reducing total operation time. Next, the circular stapler is advanced via the anus, and the descending colon is identified and checked if adequate length is available to allow a tension-free anastomosis. If necessary, the splenic flexure of the colon can be mobilized (**Figure 11**). The stapler is deployed and the donuts are checked. The pneumoperito-

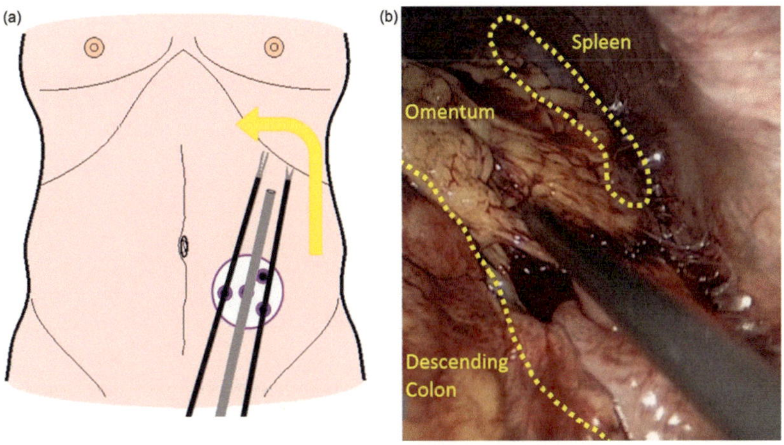

Figure 10. Adhesiolysis and mobilization of the splenic flexure.

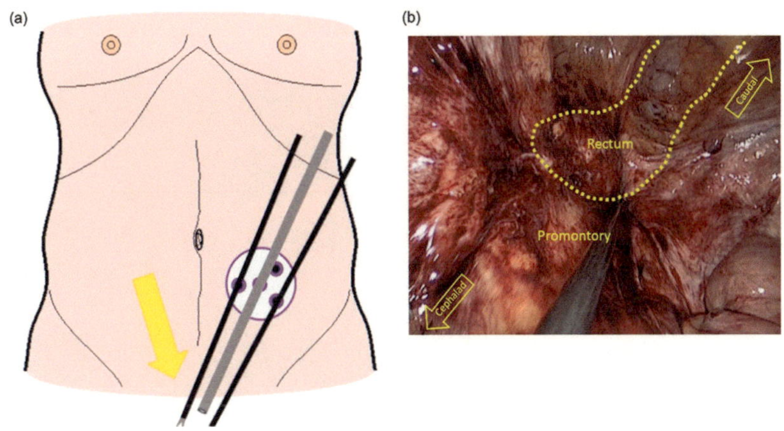

Figure 11. Dissection of adhesions and scar tissue surrounding the rectal stump.

Study	Country	Year of publication	Number of patients	Procedure	Control group (number of patients)	Morbidity (%)	Mortality (%)	Hospital stay(days)
Smith et al. [42]	USA	2011	1	Stoma site. Single port	No (0)	0(0)	0(0)	5
Carus et al. [39]	GE	2011	8	Stoma site. Single port	No (0)	1 (12.5)	0 (0)	4
Borowski et al. [38]	UK	2011	5	Stoma site. Single port	No (0)	1 (20)	0	4.2
Joshi et al. [41]	UK	2013	14	Stoma site. Glove port	No (0)	3 (21)	0 (0)	5.5
Choi et al. [40]	KR	2015	22	Stoma site. Glove port. Single port	No (0)	4 (18.2)	0(0)	8
Clermonts et al. [37]	NL	2016	25	Stoma site. Single port	Yes (16)	8 (32)	0 (0)	4

KR, Korea; NL, the Netherlands; UK, the United Kingdom; GE, Germany; USA, the United States of America.

Table 5. Summary of single-port reversal of Hartmann's procedure in the current literature.

neum is released and the trocars are removed under direct visualization. The fascia is then closed in apertures equal to or larger than 10 mm.

5.2. Appraisal of the literature

A review of the literature reveals that only a few small case series have been published on this technique. At the moment no randomized controlled trials were published [37–42]. **Table 5** summarizes the results of the available literature. The technique was first described by Smith and colleagues [42]; in this case single-port restoration of the intestinal continuity was performed in a 56-year-old patient with a history of perforated diverticulosis. Their total operation time was 104 min. The patient started a clear liquid diet on postoperative day 2 and was discharged after 5 days. The largest study without control patients was that of Choi et al. [40] and consisted of 23 patients. In one patient closure of the colostomy was aborted due to intraoperative difficulties. The median age of their patients was 62 years (range 21–87 years), with an overall ASA grade of II. Median time to reversal was 153.5 days (range 99–1028). Main indications for Hartmann's procedure were: complicated diverticulitis (27.3%), colorectal carcinoma (27.3%), and sigmoid volvulus (18.2%). They reported a median operation time of 165 minutes (range 100-340 minutes) and a total hospital stay of 8 days (range 4–31 days). There morbidity rate was 18.2% with two reoperations, one for anastomotic dehiscence and one for rectovesical fistula. No mortality was reported. Carus and colleagues' study consisted of 8 patients with a median age of 60.4 years (range 36–84). Hartmann's procedure was performed for complicated diverticulitis (five laparoscopic,

three open). The reversal was performed 2–4 months after the primary procedure. No conversions were reported in one procedure; they had to play one extra trocar had to be placed during adhesiolysis; and one patient with a superficial wound infection (morbidity 12.5%). No mortality was reported. Patients were discharged after a median of 6.4 days (range 4–8 days). The series by Clermonts et al. [37] was the only study that included a control group. They included a total of 25 patients (median age, 52.2 years). Indications for primary surgery consisted of complicated diverticulitis (60%) and malignancy in 28% of the cases. Median time to reversal was 16 months. These patients were compared with a control group in which closure of the colostomy was performed in an open method. In the open group, all primary Hartmann's procedures were performed by laparotomy; in the single-port group, 88% was performed by laparotomy. No statistical significant differences were observed between the two groups. Median operation time in the single-port group

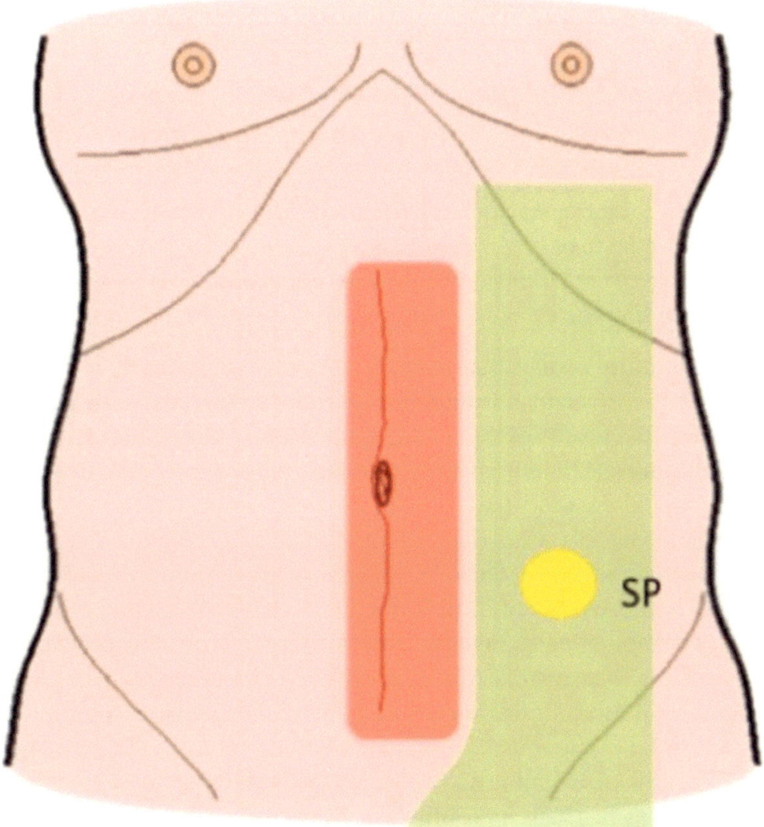

Figure 12. Port position for single-port Hartmann's reversal. SP = single-port trocar position. *Red-shaded area*: area of maximal adhesion formation after previous laparotomy. *Green-shaded area*: area of range of action that is relatively free of adhesions.

http://dx.doi.org/10.5772/66720

was 153.5 min (range: 73–332 minutes) and 184.4 min (range 29–377 minutes) in the open group. One single-port procedure was converted to laparotomy and two procedures to multiport laparoscopy due to difficulties during the adhesiolysis. In the single-port group, a total of eight complications were observed compared with 33 complications in the open group. Wound infections, 5 (20 %) versus 12 (75 %), accounted for the largest number of complications in the SPHR and OHR groups. One patient died after anastomotic leakage and sepsis in the control group; no mortality was observed in the single-port group. The median hospital stay was 4 days in the single-port group compared to a mean of 16 days in the open group.

5.3. Advantages of this technique

Single port restoration of the intestinal continuity has some major advantages over the previously mentioned techniques. The minimally invasive technique has the usual advantages of this technique with less pain and faster recovery. Specifically, in Hartmann's reversal also a shorter operation time is observed. The single port variant using the formal stoma site as an access point has the additional advantage that crossing the midline is avoided, rendering an extensive adhesiolysis unnecessary as **Figure 12** schematically shows.

Another big advantage of minimalizing the access trauma is shown in the very short hospital stay compared to the open and laparoscopic techniques. The small incision, almost no blood loss, and short operation time could be the main reasons.

6. Single-port trephine access and transanal access combined for restoration of the intestinal continuity

In Section 5 we already described the advantages of single-port restoration of intestinal continuity with access through the formal site of the colostomy. Recently, a new technique that combines the single-port trephine access with single-port transanal access was presented [43]. It is suggested the transanal approach will aid in the technically challenging dissection of the rectal stump and perform a pelvic adhesiolysis in a safer manner.

6.1. Surgical technique

Patients receive mechanical bowel and rectal stump cleansing. Patients are placed in lithotomy position. The procedure is performed by two surgeons starting simultaneously; one surgeon starts the abdominal trephine access approach (Section 5). The second surgeon places a single-port transanal access platform through the anal canal with three working trocars. The pneumorectum is created. Next, circular dissection next to the stapler line in the proximal part of the rectal stump is performed into the avascular presacral plane posteriorly. This plane of dissection is extended medially, laterally, and interiorly to achieve the desired circumferential rectal mobilization. Finally, the peritoneal reflection

was visualized and divided to achieve the proximal rectal stump removal, with both surgeons working together. The previous stapler line with the resected tissue can be extracted transanally. Next, a Prolene purse-string suture is used to close the distal rectal stump. In order to complete the end-to-end anastomosis, a circular stapler is inserted via the anal canal and connected to the anvil in the proximal descending colon. After firing the circular stapler and completing the anastomosis, the integrity of the anastomosis can be evaluated with an air test, as well as an intraluminal examination through the transanal access platform.

6.2. Critical appraisal of literature

A review of the literature reveals one study by Bravo and colleagues [43]. The study group describes a technique that is easily adopted and mastered by surgeons already trained in transanal colorectal surgery. They report no postoperative morbidity and a quick recovery and discharge from the hospital (no exact numbers given). Furthermore, a shorter total operation time is mentioned when compared to a multiport laparoscopic approach.

Advantages of this technique mentioned by the authors are first of all the safe dissection of the rectal stump because most of the work is done in a surgical plane not touched during the initial surgery and thus without adhesions. This gives the ability to precisely identify structures with adherence to the rectal stump like small bowel or ureter. The main difficulty of this technique can be performing the transanal dissection in patients with hard adhesions to the rectal stump after perforation or peritonitis. Furthermore, a very short rectal stump makes positioning the transanal single-port access difficult and without adequate workspace impossible.

7. Authors' recommendation

The authors believe that the minimally invasive technique is an attractive approach for rever-sal of Hartmann's procedure. So far, reports are promising. The technique may reduce the substantial morbidity known from open reversal. The SIR technique may be considered to be obsolete, especially in the era of laparoscopy. Most patients will be best suited by use of lapa-roscopic techniques. We would like to emphasize that laparoscopy is a means to an end and not a goal in itself. If minimally invasive techniques are deemed unsafe or unsuitable, conver-sion to open technique may be utilized at any time. We believe that. The recently developed technique of single port restoration of continuity seems especially promising, as contralateral access that can be cumbersome due to the adhesions from a previous laparotomy is avoided and a ventral hernia defect when present can be avoided. We believe Trephine assess in combination with the transanal approach as primary surgical approach is not always necessary. We recommend this technique to be used as a step-up approach or back-up when pelvic dissection is proving technically challenging

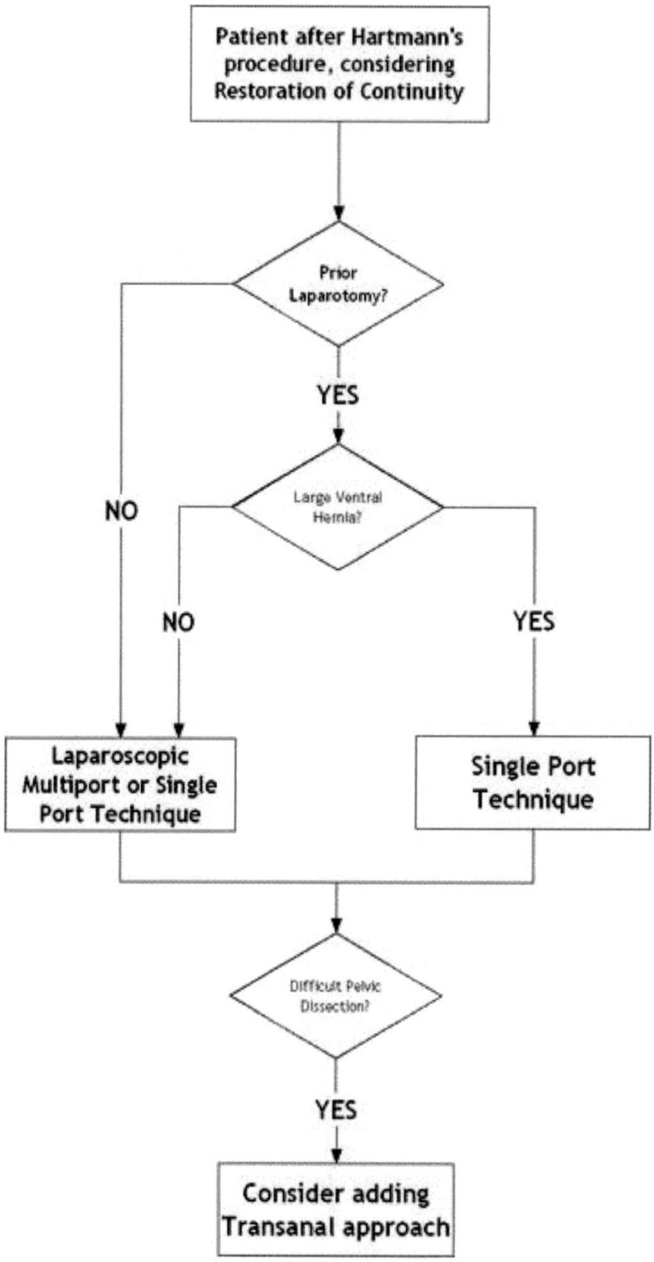

Figure 13. Algorithm to be used during the decision-making which technique is best suited for the restoration of bowel continuity after Hartmann's procedure.

or unsafe during initial trephine or multiport access. Authors recommendations are summarized in the algorithm in **Figure 13**.

8. Conclusion

The reversal of Hartmann's procedure carries a high operative morbidity and mortality rate. Therefore this is only performed in a selected group of patients. A considerable group of patients, with advanced age, or expected high operative risk, are left with a permanent end colostomy. This chapter gives an overview of the development less invasive techniques, that may reduce morbidity and therefore be offered to a larger group of patients.

Conventional laparoscopic reversal of Hartmann's procedure was the first technique with the primary goal of reducing morbidity and mortally. This technique reduced surgical access trauma resulting in a shorter post operative hospital stay and avoiding the negative consequences of relaparotomy. In the quest for even less invasive ways of restoring the bowel continuity the Trephine access technique was developed. This technique received criticism on the fact that the adhesiolysis was performed mainly in a blind fashion. This is probably the reason why this technique has not gained wide popularity and acceptance. This technique however gave birth to the development of the single-port access technique. This minimally invasive laparoscopic technique has our preference. We recommend using this technique for the major reduction in access trauma. Avoiding crossing the midline reduces the need for adhesiolysis, with its potential hazards like iatrogenic bowel injury. When proven safe in larger series, reversal of Hartmann's procedure may be offered to a larger proportion of patients then is presently routine.

Author details

Stefan H.E.M. Clermonts[1], Laurents P.S. Stassen[2] and David D.E. Zimmerman[1,*]

*Address all correspondence to: d.zimmerman@etz.nl

1 Department of Surgery, Elisabeth-TweeSteden Hospital, Tilburg, The Netherlands

2 Department of Surgery, Maastricht University Medical Center, Maastricht, The Netherlands

References

[1] Van Gulik TM, Mallonga ET, Taat CW. Henri Hartmann, Lord of the Hotel-Dieu. Nether J Surg. 1986(3):45–7.

[2] JP. Portraits de Chirurgiens de l'Hotel-Dieu. Presse Med. 1959(60):2317–20.

[3] Ronel DN, Hardy MA. Henri Albert Hartmann: labor and discipline. Curr Surg. 2002;59(1):59–64.

[4] HH. Nouveau procede d'ablation des cancers de la partie terminale du colon pelvien. Strasbourg: Trentienne Congres de Chirurgie, 1921:411–3.

[5] HH. Note sur un procede nouveau d'extripation des cancers de la partie terminale du colon. Bulletin et Memoires de la Societe Chirurgique de Paris. 1923:1474–7.

[6] Abbas S. Resection and primary anastomosis in acute complicated diverticulitis, a systematic review of the literature. Int J Colorectal Dis. 2007;22(4):351–7.

[7] Pearce NW, Scott SD, Karran SJ. Timing and method of reversal of Hartmann's procedure. Br J Surg. 1992;79(8):839–41.

[8] Wigmore SJ, Duthie GS, Young IE, Spalding EM, Rainey JB. Restoration of intestinal continuity following Hartmann's procedure: the Lothian experience 1987–1992. Br J Surg. 1995;82(1):27–30.

[9] Albarran SA, Simoens C, Van De Winkel N, da Costa PM, Thill V. Restoration of digestive continuity after Hartmann's procedure: ASA score is a predictive factor for risk of postoperative complications. Acta Chir Belg. 2009;109(6):714–9.

[10] Banerjee S, Leather AJ, Rennie JA, Samano N, Gonzalez JG, Papagrigoriadis S. Feasibility and morbidity of reversal of Hartmann's. Colorectal Dis: Off J Assoc Coloproctol G B Irel. 2005;7(5):454–9.

[11] Maggard MA, Zingmond D, O'Connell JB, Ko CY. What proportion of patients with an ostomy (for diverticulitis) get reversed? Am Surg. 2004;70(10):928–31.

[12] Nugent KP, Daniels P, Stewart B, Patankar R, Johnson CD. Quality of life in stoma patients. Dis Colon Rectum. 1999;42(12):1569–74.

[13] Mols F, Lemmens V, Bosscha K, van den Broek W, Thong MS. Living with the physicaland mental consequences of an ostomy: a study among 1-10-year rectal cancer survivorsfrom the population-based PROFILES registry. Psychooncology. 2014. Sep;23(9):998–1004.

[14] Roque-Castellano C, Marchena-Gomez J, Hemmersbach-Miller M, Acosta-Merida A, Rodriguez-Mendez A, Farina-Castro R, et al. Analysis of the factors related to the decision of restoring intestinal continuity after Hartmann's procedure. Int J Colorectal Dis. 2007;22(9):1091–6.

[15] Machairas A, Liakakos T, Patapis P, Petropoulos C, Tsapralis D, Misiakos EP. Prosthetic repair of incisional hernia combined with elective bowel operation. Surgeon: J R Coll Surg Edinb Irel. 2008;6(5):274–7.

[16] Seo SI, Lee JL, Park SH, Ha HK, Kim JC. Assessment by using a water-soluble contrast enema study of radiologic leakage in lower rectal cancer patients with sphincter-saving surgery. Ann Coloproctol. 2015;31(4):131–7.

[17] Kalady MF, Mantyh CR, Petrofski J, Ludwig KA. Routine contrast imaging of low pelvic anastomosis prior to closure of defunctioning ileostomy: is it necessary? J Gastrointest Surg. 2008;12(7):1227–31.

[18] Hong SY, Kim do Y, Oh SY, Suh KW. Routine barium enema prior to closure of defunctioning ileostomy is not necessary. J Korean Surg Soc. 2012;83(2):88–91.

[19] Keck JO, Collopy BT, Ryan PJ, Fink R, Mackay JR, Woods RJ. Reversal of Hartmann's procedure: effect of timing and technique on ease and safety. Dis Colon Rectum. 1994;37(3):243–8.

[20] Roe AM, Prabhu S, Ali A, Brown C, Brodribb AJ. Reversal of Hartmann's procedure: timing and operative technique. Br J Surg. 1991;78(10):1167–70.

[21] Kwon S, Morris A, Billingham R, Frankhouse J, Horvath K, Johnson M, et al. Routine leak testing in colorectal surgery in the Surgical Care and Outcomes Assessment Program. Arch Surg. 2012;147(4):345–51.

[22] Aydin HN, Remzi FH, Tekkis PP, Fazio VW. Hartmann's reversal is associated with high postoperative adverse events. Dis Colon Rectum. 2005;48(11):2117–26.

[23] Carcoforo P, Navarra G, Di Marco L, Occhionorelli S, Rocca T, Pollinzi V. Reversal of Hartmann's procedure. Our experience. Ann Ital Chir. 1997;68(4):523–7; discussion 7–8.

[24] Rosen MJ, Cobb WS, Kercher KW, Sing RF, Heniford BT. Laparoscopic restoration of intestinal continuity after Hartmann's procedure. Am J Surg. 2005;189(6):670–4.

[25] Faure JP, Doucet C, Essique D, Badra Y, Carretier M, Richer JP, et al. Comparison of conventional and laparoscopic Hartmann's procedure reversal. Surg Laparosc Endosc Percutan Tech. 2007;17(6):495–9.

[26] Haughn C, Ju B, Uchal M, Arnaud JP, Reed JF, Bergamaschi R. Complication rates after Hartmann's reversal: open vs. laparoscopic approach. Dis Colon Rectum. 2008;51(8):1232–6.

[27] Vermeulen J, Coene PP, Van Hout NM, van der Harst E, Gosselink MP, Mannaerts GH, et al. Restoration of bowel continuity after surgery for acute perforated diverticulitis: should Hartmann's procedure be considered a one-stage procedure? Colorectal Dis. 2009;11(6):619–24.

[28] Mazeh H, Greenstein AJ, Swedish K, Nguyen SQ, Lipskar A, Weber KJ, et al. Laparoscopic and open reversal of Hartmann's procedure—a comparative retrospective analysis. Surg Endosc. 2009;23(3):496–502.

[29] Di Carlo I, Toro A, Pannofino O, Patane E, Pulvirenti E. Laparoscopic versus open restoration of intestinal continuity after Hartmann procedure. Hepatogastroenterology. 2010;57(98):232–5.

[30] De'angelis N, Brunetti F, Memeo R, Batista da Costa J, Schneck AS, Carra MC, et al. Comparison between open and laparoscopic reversal of Hartmann's procedure for diverticulitis. World J Gastrointest Surg. 2013;5(8):245–51.

[31] Yang PF, Morgan MJ. Laparoscopic versus open reversal of Hartmann's procedure: a retrospective review. ANZ J Surg. 2014;84(12):965–9.

[32] Vermeulen J VW, Mannaerts GH, . Reversal of Hartmann's procedure through the stomal side: a new even more minimal invasive technique. Surg Endosc 2008;22(10):2319–22.

[33] van de Wall BJ, Draaisma WA, Schouten ES, Broeders IA, Consten EC. Conventional and laparoscopic reversal of the Hartmann procedure: a review of literature. J Gastrointest Surg. 2010;14(4):743–52.

[34] Vermeulen J., LJWA, Mannaerts GHH. Reversal of Hartmann's procedure after perforated diverticulitis through the stomal side without additional incisions: the SIR procedure. Dig Surg. 2010;27:391–6.

[35] Aydin C, Olmez A, Isik S, Sumer F, Kayaalp C. Reversal of the Hartmann procedure through only a stomal orifice. Am Surg. 2011;77(6):694–6.

[36] Parkin E, Khurshid M, Ravi S, Linn T. Surgical access through the stoma for laparoscopic reversal of Hartmann procedures. Surg Laparosc Endosc Percutan Tech. 2013;23(1):41–4.

[37] Clermonts SH, de Ruijter WM, van Loon YT, Wasowicz DK, Heisterkamp J, Maring JK, et al. Reversal of Hartmann's procedure utilizing single-port laparoscopy: an attractive alternative to laparotomy. Surg Endosc. 2016;30(5):1894–901.

[38] Borowski DW, Kanakala V, Agarwal AK, Tabaqchali MA, Garg DK, Gill TS. Single-port access laparoscopic reversal of Hartmann operation. Dis Colon Rectum. 2011;54(8):1053–6.

[39] Carus T, Emmert A. Single-port laparoscopic reversal of Hartmann's procedure: technique and results. Minim Invasive Surg 2011;2011:356784.

[40] Choi BJ, Jeong WJ, Kim YK, Kim SJ, Lee SC. Single-port laparoscopic reversal of Hartmann's procedure via the colostomy site. Int J Surg 2015;14:33–7.

[41] Joshi HM, Gosselink MP, Adusumilli S, Cunningham C, Lindsey I, Jones OM. Incisionless reversal of Hartmann's procedure. Tech Coloproctol. 2014;18(9):843–6.

[42] Smith BM, Bettinger DA. Single-incision laparoscopic reversal of Hartmann procedure via the colostomy site only: first report. Surg Innov. 2011;18(4):NP5–7.

[43] Bravo R, Fernandez-Hevia M, Jimenez-Toscano M, Flores LF, de Lacy B, Quaresima S, et al. Transanal Hartmann reversal: a new technique. Surg Endosc. 2016;30(6):2628–31.

Chapter 2

Bariatric and Metabolic Surgery

Chih Kun Huang, Sir Emmanuel S. Astudillo,
Prasad M. Bhukebag and Khan Wei Chan

Additional information is available at the end of the chapter

http://dx.doi.org/10.5772/107288

Abstract

Obesity as a global epidemic has rapidly increased in incidence in the recent few decades and represents one of the biggest public health challenges. Obesity plays a major risk for various diseases such as cardiovascular disease (CVD), diabetes mellitus (DM), hypercholesterolemia, osteoarthritis and some form of cancers. Bariatric and metabolic surgery provides the best solution for obesity and its associated comorbidities. This chapter will discuss in detail the commonly performed bariatric and metabolic surgeries.

Keywords: bariatric surgery, metabolic surgery, Roux-en-Y gastric bypass, sleeve gastrectomy, duodenojejunal bypass, proximal jejunal bypass, obesity, type 2 diabetes

1. Introduction

Bariatric surgery has been established to be the most effective treatment for morbid obesity, producing sustained and durable weight loss with improvement or remission of comorbidities and longer life [1]. The procedures undertaken to treat morbid obesity have changed over a period of time and recently newer procedures are being developed with lesser morbidity and mortality and better results. The resolution of comorbidities such as type 2 diabetes mellitus (T2DM), hypertension and others after bariatric surgery gave impetus to the concept of metabolic surgery. Metabolic surgery has become increasingly effective and accepted option for patients with T2DM [2]. This chapter will describe in detail two most commonly performed procedures, laparoscopic sleeve gastrectomy (LSG) and laparoscopic Roux-en-Y gastric bypass (LRYGB). Part of the chapter also details the sleeve gastrectomy-based procedures which include sleeve gastrectomy with loop duodenojejunal bypass (LDJB-SG) and sleeve gastrectomy with proximal jejunal bypass (SG-PJB).

2. Laparoscopic sleeve gastrectomy

Laparoscopic Sleeve Gastrectomy (LSG) or "sleeve" is now one of the most commonly performed bariatric procedures worldwide. It is a purely restrictive procedure without intestinal bypass. In 1999, Michel Gagner and his team performed the first laparoscopic duodenal switch on the porcine model and found it to be feasible. Laparoscopic duodenal switch was later performed in morbid obese patients and found to have higher morbidity in higher BMI patients. Staged procedure was then undertaken to reduce the mortality and morbidity with laparoscopic sleeve gastrectomy as the first stage of a two-stage duodenal switch. However, the initial weight loss after LSG alone was found to be adequate and maintained over a period of time. The second stage of surgery was deferred or was not required at all and patients maintained good weight loss with just the first stage. After this success and some modifications to the procedure, sleeve gastrectomy was established as an effective stand-alone bariatric procedure.

Apart from restriction of size of stomach, reduction in the "hunger hormone" ghrelin, after LSG decreases appetite. Advantages of LSG include lower operative complexity, relative safety and maintenance of pylorus and easy convertibility to other procedures. Also, since there are no bowel bypass problems of internal herniation, small bowel obstruction, micronutrient deficiencies and malnutrition will not be encountered.

The disadvantages of the procedure include irreversibility, possibility of staple line leak, bleeding and stricture of gastric tube. The incidence of gastroesophageal reflux has also been found to be increased in some patients undergoing this procedure.

2.1. Indications and contraindications

Indications for this procedure include BMI ≥ 40 kg/m^2 without comorbidities or ≥35 kg/m^2 with comorbidities. This can also be offered as a first stage of biliopancreatic diversion in patients with BMI > 50 kg/m^2. Contraindications include chronic alcoholism, drug and substance abuse, major psychiatric disorder, severe gastroesophageal reflux disease and chronic duodenal ulcer.

2.2. Preoperative work up and preparation

Comprehensive preoperative workup for sleeve gastrectomy is the same as that of the other bariatric procedures. Patients are admitted the day prior to the procedure when they are started on clear liquid diet. Single dose of prophylactic antibiotic and proton pump inhibitor are given an hour prior to surgery. Low molecular-weight heparin (LMWH) is prescribed to lower the incidence of deep vein thrombosis (DVT) and other thromboembolic events, till the patient is ambulated.

2.3. Operative technique

2.3.1. Positioning

Patient is positioned flat on the operating table with both upper extremities extended out. Patient is secured at the chest and thighs using straps and a foot board in preparation for a steep reverse Trendelenburg position. The surgeon and the scrub nurse both stand on the patient's right while the first assistant and the cameraman stand on the patient's left.

http://dx.doi.org/10.5772/107288

2.3.2. Port placement

A three-four ports technique is utilized for this procedure as shown in **Figure 1**. Pneumoperitoneum is created by Veress needle or optical trocar is used at the first port. The first port is about three finger breadths to the left of umbilicus, at about 20 cm from the xiphisternum. The second 15 mm port is inserted at supraumbilical site. Another 5 mm trocar is inserted in the right midclavicular line below the costal margin, for surgeon's left hand, such that the falciform ligament does not cause difficulty in dissection of the hiatus. Lastly an optional 5 mm assistant port can be placed in the left anterior axillary line just below the costal margin.

2.3.3. Placement of liver suspension tape

To elevate the central and left lobe of the liver, a liver suspension tape (LST) was designed. Two pieces of Jackson-Pratt (JP) drain measuring 2 cm each were cut and fixed with 2/0 polypropylene suture (Ethicon W8400 2-0 Prolene blue 70 mm round bodied). The lateral segment of the left lobe was suspended using the tape by passing the needle through the liver, out through the anterior abdominal wall and secured with clamps. Another LST was inserted in the medial aspect of left lobe of liver to retract the liver completely.

The LSTs should not be placed more than 2 cm away from the liver edge to achieve optimal retraction and prevent major bile duct or vessel injury (**Figure 2**). Alternatively, a Nathanson

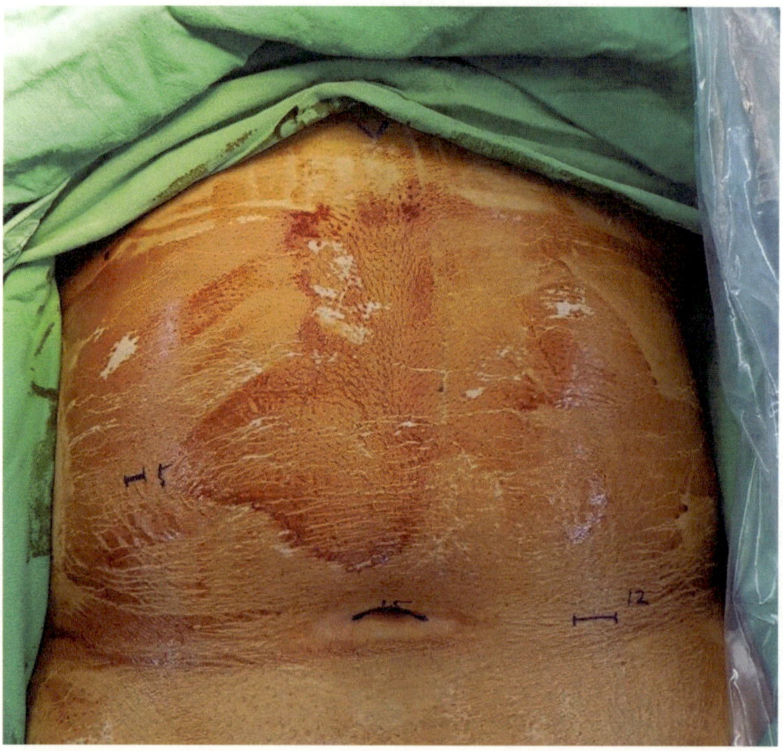

Figure 1. Port placement for LSG.

liver retractor (C-NLRS-1001 Cook Medical) may be used in order to achieve good exposure of the entire length of the stomach and duodenum. This may be placed using a 5 mm port inserted in the subxiphoid area.

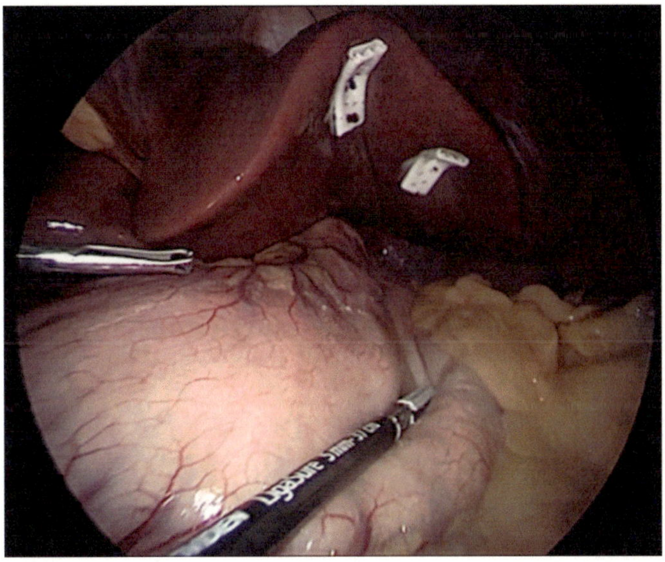

Figure 2. Retraction of left lobe of liver with liver suspension tape.

2.3.4. Mobilization of the gastrocolic ligament

Dissection of the gastrocolic ligament close to the greater curvature of the stomach commences at a point opposite the incisura angularis. A window in the lesser sac is created and dissection is started using a vessel sealing energy device (Ligasure™ vessel sealing device by Covidien-Medtronic or Harmonic Ace by Ethicon). By staying very close to the gastric wall, the entire gastrocolic ligament is detached up to the angle of His taking care at the area of the short gastric vessels at the splenic hilum (**Figures 3** and **4**). Care should be taken not to injure left gastric vessels.

2.3.5. Dissection at the angle of His

Fundus of the stomach must be mobilized from its adhesions and completely resected. A very useful anatomical landmark is to expose the left crus of the hiatus. Dissection of the left crus is terminated once the left phrenoesophageal ligament has been completely visualized (**Figure 5**). The posterior attachments of the fundus to the anterior border of the pancreas are completely mobilized to properly identify and preserve the left gastric vessels (**Figure 6**).

The anterior portion of the gastroesophageal fat pad (Belsey's pad of fat) is then dissected in order to expose half of the anterior portion of the GE junction. Care is taken not to completely devascularize this fat pad which may increase the rate of leak at the GE junction.

http://dx.doi.org/10.5772/107288

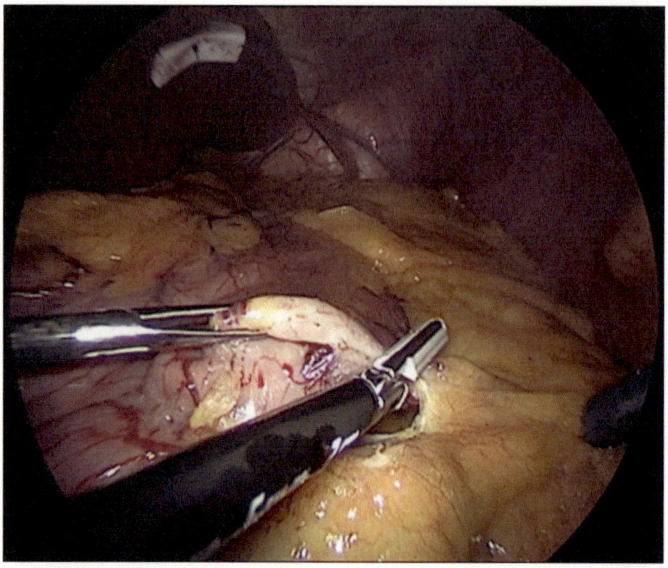

Figure 3. Start of dissection by creating a window in the lesser sac.

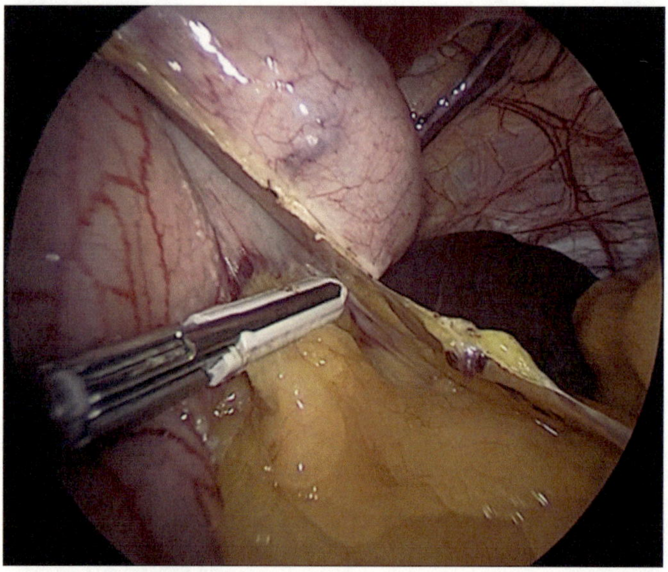

Figure 4. Dissection of the gastrocolic ligament at short gastric vessels near splenic hilum.

2.3.6. Dissection of the caudal part of the gastrocolic ligament

The gastrocolic ligament at the area of the right gastroepiploic vessel is dissected caudally till the distance of 4 cm from the pylorus. Dense adhesions around the prepyloric area may be encountered and should be taken down individually (**Figure 7**).

2.3.7. Sleeve gastrectomy

Prior to the creation of the actual sleeve, make sure that the entire stomach is laid down flat. At this point, the anesthesiologist inserts an orogastric tube with its tip positioned by the surgeon under direct visual guidance. Using an L-hook dissector (STORZ 37370DL Monopolar Dissecting L-Hook Cannula), marking on the anterior surface of the stomach is done which

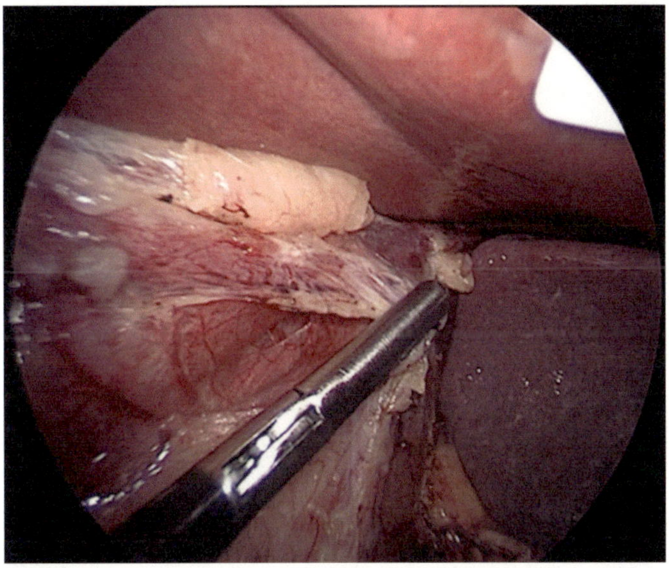

Figure 5. Dissection at the angle of His exposing the left crus and phrenoesophageal ligament.

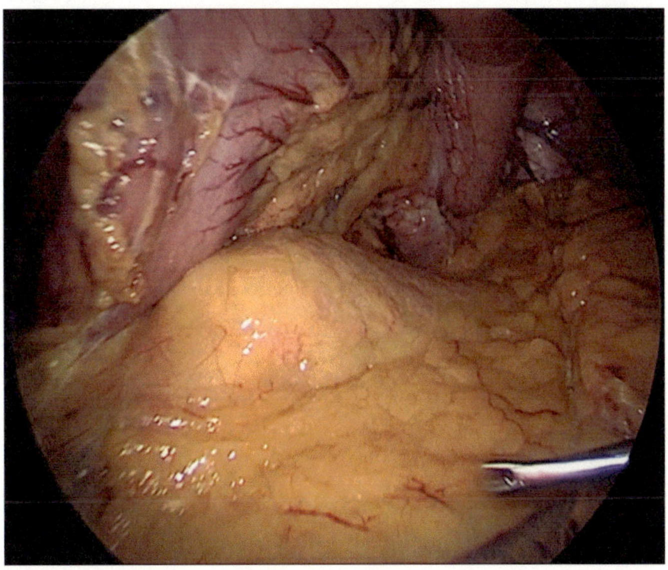

Figure 6. Complete mobilization of the posterior attachments of the fundus and anterior border of the pancreas.

http://dx.doi.org/10.5772/107288

will serve as a guide for the surgeon to place the endostapler with 38 Fr orogastric tube as stent (**Figure 8**). For the first staple firing, the stapling device is placed 4 cm away from the pylorus and 2.5–3 cm away from the incisura angularis in order to prevent narrowing (**Figure 9**). A black 60 mm reload (EGIA60AXT Endo GIA 60 mm articulating extra-thick reload with Tri-Staple Technology) or a green 60 mm green reload (ECR60G Echelon Endopath stapler reload cartridges by Ethicon) using manual or powered device is used. Successive firings

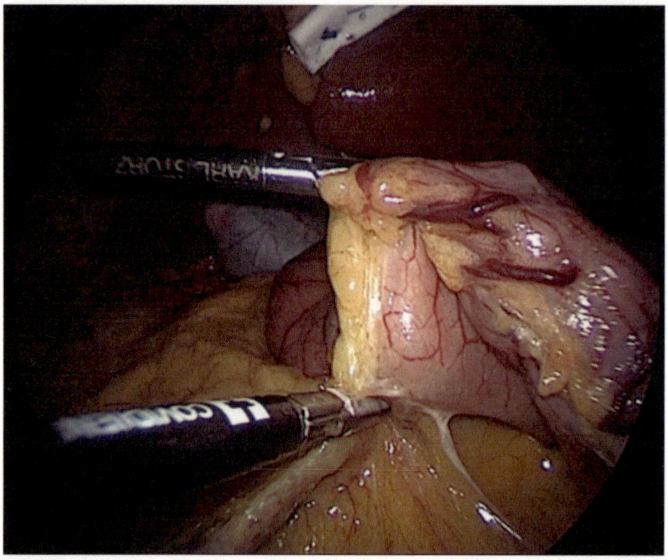

Figure 7. Dissection of the gastrocolic ligament toward the pylorus.

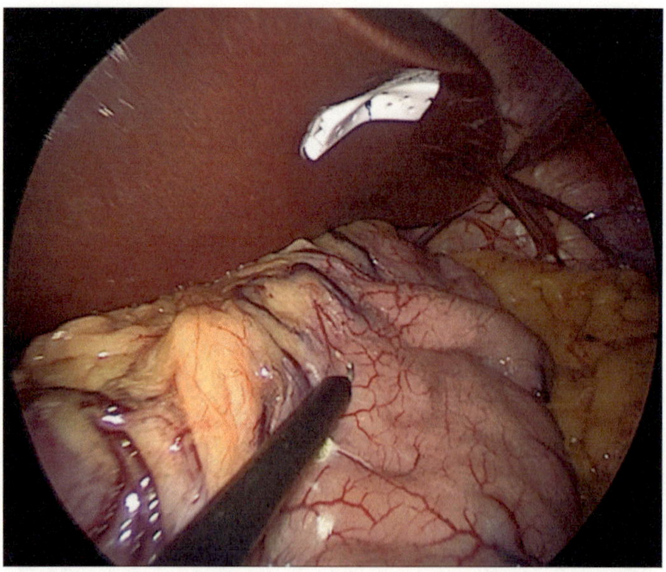

Figure 8. Marking of the transection line along the anterior surface of the stomach.

of the stapling device toward the gastric fundus are done using either a 60 mm purple cartridge (EGIA60AMT Endo GIA 60 mm articulating medium/thick reload with Tri-Staple Technology) or a 60 mm blue cartridge (ETHECR60B Echelon Endopath stapler reload cartridges by Ethicon) (**Figure 10**). Commencing after placement of the second stapler, loose migratory crotch staples must be removed in order to prevent improper formation of the

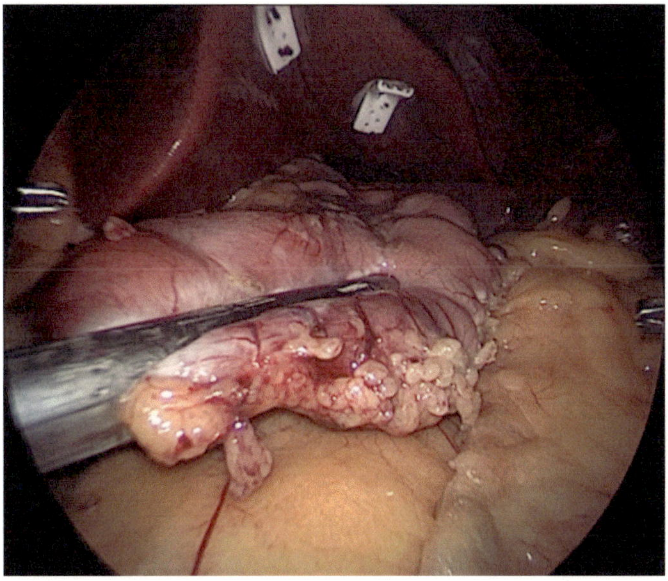

Figure 9. First staple firing 4 cm from pylorus and 2.5–3 cm away from the incisura.

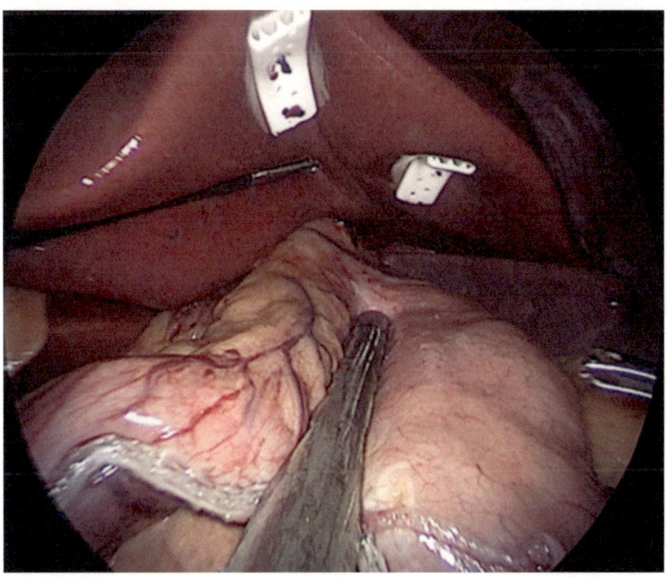

Figure 10. Successive firings of the staple device toward the fundus.

http://dx.doi.org/10.5772/107288

suture line (**Figure 11**). Constant communication with the anesthesiologist is of paramount importance, inserting and withdrawing the orogastric tube before and after application of each stapler to make sure the bougie is not stapled into the remnant stomach. It is also highly recommended to check the posterior aspect of the stomach before each firing of the device in order to avoid twisting and in-folding of tissues. The entire fundus, including its posterior

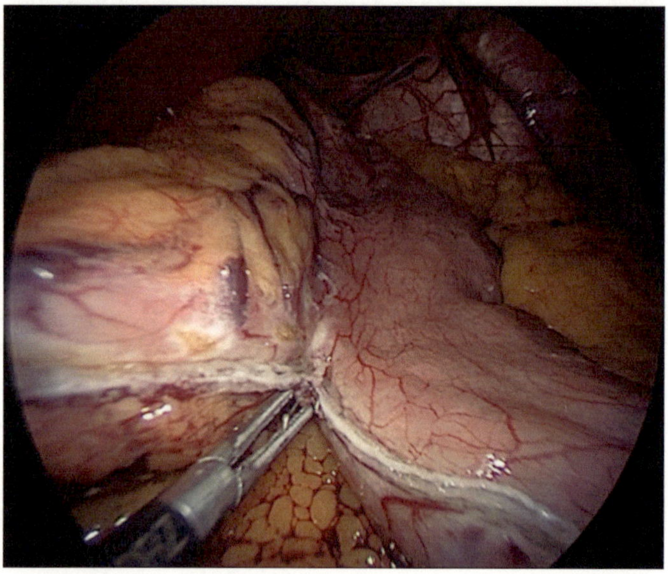

Figure 11. Removal of migratory crotch staples.

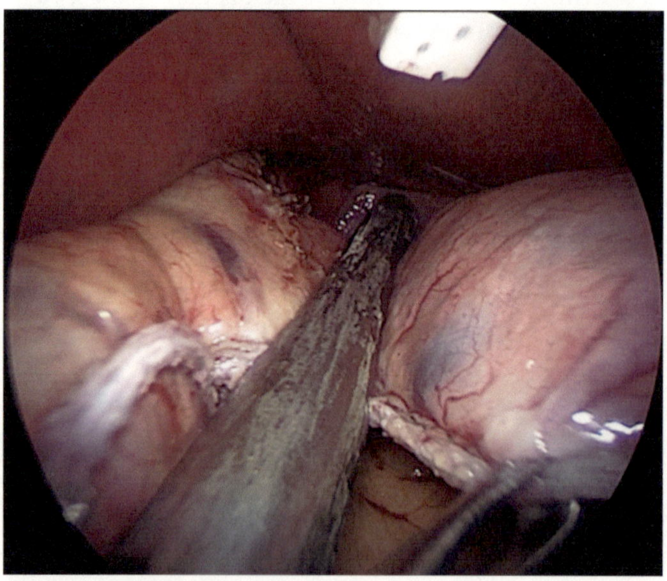

Figure 12. Staple firing 1 cm away from the GE junction.

wall, is to be included in the resected part. Before firing of the last stapler, always verify that the stapler is placed not less than 1 cm from the GE junction and that both tips of the stapler are always in sight (**Figure 12**).

2.3.8. Hemostasis

The entire length of the staple line should be inspected for any bleeding. Bleeding may be controlled using electrocautery, clips or over sewing. No buttressing material is placed over the staple line.

2.3.9. Fixing the tube

One or two fixing stitches are taken between the stapled sleeve and the retroperitoneal fat to prevent rotation of the sleeve tube.

2.3.10. Specimen extraction

The LSTs are removed and the entry and exit points on the liver are cauterized to achieve hemostasis. Specimen is then extracted through the umbilical port and closure of the rectus sheath done with 2-0 Vicryl. Subcutaneous layers of all ports closed with 3-0 Vicryl and skin closed with interrupted subcuticular stitches. Dermabond is applied and dressing done.

2.3.11. Surgical outcomes

The mechanism of action of LSG appears to be by the restriction of the volume of stomach and the removal of ghrelin-producing fundus [3]. The decreased ghrelin leads to early satiety and decreased hunger. Another mechanism is increased gastric emptying which combined with decreased gastric acid secretion causes incomplete digestion [4]. Increased gastric emptying is associated with higher levels of glucagon-like-peptide-1 (GLP-1), a glucose-regulating insulin-enhancing agent, which has been linked to weight loss and resolution of type 2 diabetes mellitus [5].

In a retrospective study, the EWL after 3 and 6 years follow-up of LSG was 72.8 and 57.3%, respectively [4]. Gustavo et al. in their long-term study showed a mean %EBMIL (percentage of excess BMI Loss) of 82.4, 75.9 and 62.5 and % TWL (percentage of total weight loss) of 28.5, 25.8 and 21 at 3, 6 and 11+ years of follow-up, respectively [6].

3. Sleeve-based procedures

One of the arguments against LSG is that its weight loss as well as its efficacy in diabetes remission is inferior and not sustainable compared to RYGB. This is owed to the fact that LSG do not own the content of bowel bypass. Laparoscopic loop duodenojejunal bypass with sleeve gastrectomy (LDJB-SG) and sleeve gastrectomy with proximal jejunal bypass (SG-PJB) are a combination of both a restrictive and malabsorptive procedures (**Figure 13** and **28**). First described by Huang et al. in 2011, LDJB-SG has a lower incidence of dumping syndrome and marginal ulcer, both commonly experienced in RYGB, due to an intact pylorus which acts as

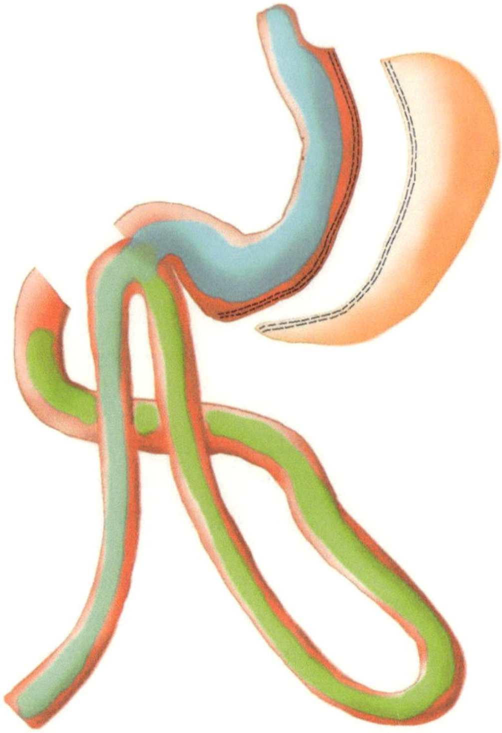

Figure 13. Schematic diagram of LDJB-SG.

a sphincter mechanism and a creates a neutral condition from mixture of gastric acid, pancreatic juice and bile around the duodenojejunal anastomosis [7]. SG-PJB was designed by Alamo et al. in 2005 and later revised in 2009 [9, 10]. Surgical results of weight loss and comorbidity resolution were comparable to Roux-en-Y gastric bypass in his reports. Both LDJB-SG and SGPJB can be an alternative operation that could potentially lessen the complications associated with the conventional gastric bypass.

3.1. Loop DuodenoJejunal Bypass with Sleeve Gastrectomy

3.1.1. Indications and Contraindications

Indication for this procedure includes BMI ≥ 40 kg/m^2 without comorbidities or ≥35 kg/m^2. This can also be offered as a surgical treatment for poorly controlled type 2 diabetes in Asian patients with BMI ≥ 32.5 kg/m^2 without comorbidities or >27.5 kg/m^2 with comorbidities. Contraindications include chronic alcoholism, drug and substance abuse, major psychiatric disorder, severe gastroesophageal reflux disease and chronic duodenal ulcer [8].

3.1.2. Preoperative work up and preparation

Comprehensive preoperative workup for DJB-SG is the same as that of the other bariatric procedures. Patients are admitted the day prior to the procedure were they are started on clear liquid diet. Single dose of prophylactic antibiotic and proton pump inhibitor are given

an hour prior to surgery. Low molecular-weight heparin (LMWH) is prescribed to lower the incidence of deep vein thrombosis (DVT) and other thromboembolic events.

3.1.3. *Positioning*

Patient is positioned flat on the operating table with both upper extremities extended out. Patient is secured at the chest and thighs using straps and a foot board in preparation for a steep reverse Trendelenburg position. The surgeon and the scrub nurse both stand on the patient's right while the first assistant and the cameraman stand on the patient's left.

3.1.4. *Operative Technique*

3.1.4.1. *Port placement*

Five-port technique is utilized for this procedure as shown in **Figure 14**. A 12 mm optical port on the left of umbilicus is placed after abdominal cavity is entered using the closed Veress technique or via an optical trocar. One 15 mm port is placed in immediate supraumbilical region and another 12 mm port is placed to the right of umbilicus mirroring the one on the left, both of which serve as the surgeon's right hand working ports. A 5 mm trocar is placed in the right midclavicular line below the costal margin for the surgeon's left hand while another 5 mm trocar is placed in the midclavicular line below the left subcostal margin for the assistant.

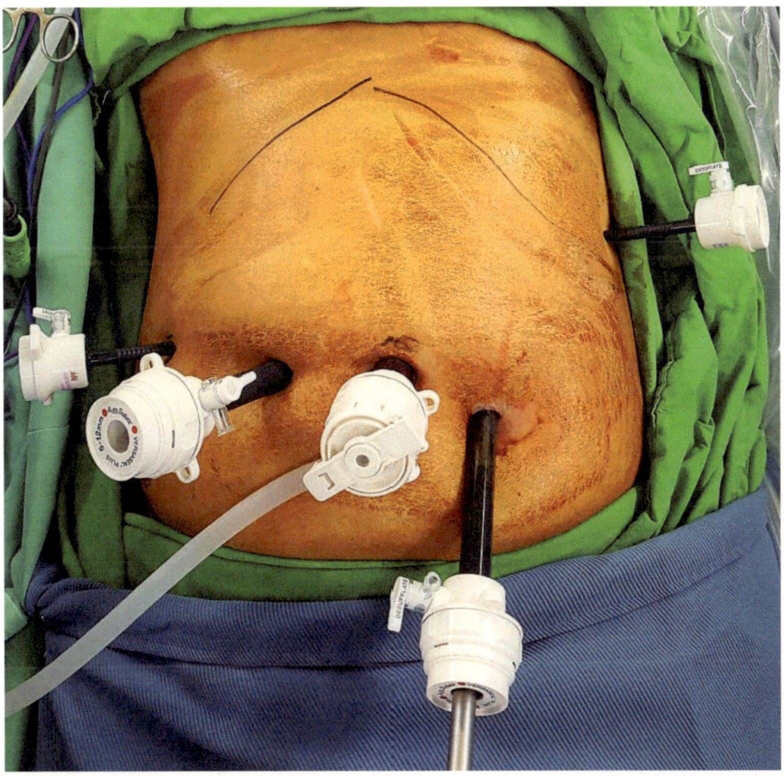

Figure 14. Port placement for LDJB-SG.

http://dx.doi.org/10.5772/107288

3.1.4.2. Placement of liver suspension tape

An LST previously discussed earlier in this chapter is utilized. However, instead of using a 2.5 cm cut JP drain, 5 cm is used for the second tape in order to lift both the lobes of the liver along with the falciform ligament away from the field (**Figure 15**).

3.1.4.3. Sleeve gastrectomy

The formation of the gastric sleeve tube is done in a similar way as described earlier in this chapter.

3.1.4.4. Duodenal transection

Proper exposure of the entire length of the stomach and first part of the duodenum is critical to the success of this procedure. After sleeve gastrectomy has been performed, the next step is to dissect the first part of the duodenum. A counter traction suture is placed at the distal end of the sleeved stomach to visualize the first part of the duodenum (**Figure 16**). At a distance approximately 2 cm distal to the pylorus, a tunnel is created posterior to the duodenal wall and just anterior to the gastroduodenal artery using a combination of a blunt dissector and Flexlap Gold Finger retractor (Flexlap Gold Finger Retractor by Ethicon Endo Surgery, USA) as seen in **Figures 17** and **18**. A tape is then passed in the tunnel behind the duodenum and lifted laterally and downwards to serve as a traction while inserting the endostapler (**Figure 19**). Using a 45 mm curved tip articulating tan reload (EGIA45CTAVM Endo GIA 45 mm Curved Tip articulating vascular/medium reload with Tri-Staple™ Technology), the first part of the duodenum is transected. Care is taken to avoid injury to the common bile duct (CBD), pancreas and major vessels in the area (**Figure 20**) [8].

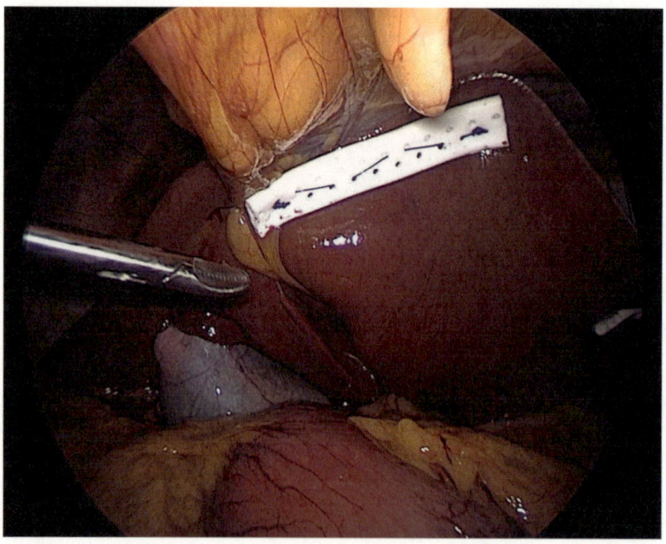

Figure 15. Liver suspension for both lobes.

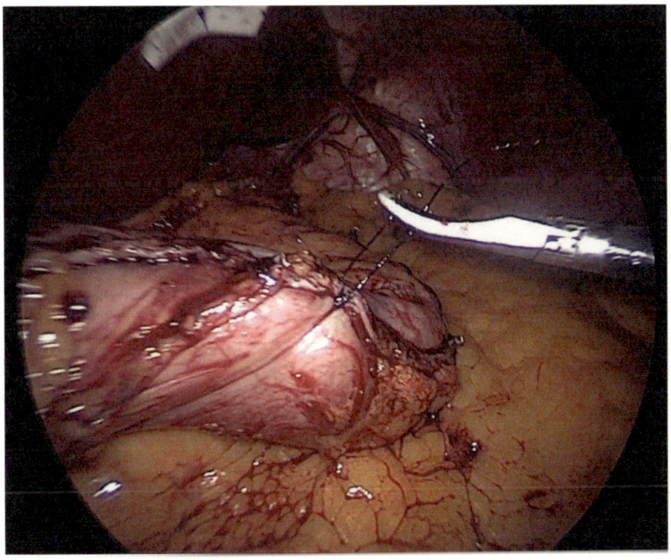

Figure 16. Counter traction suture.

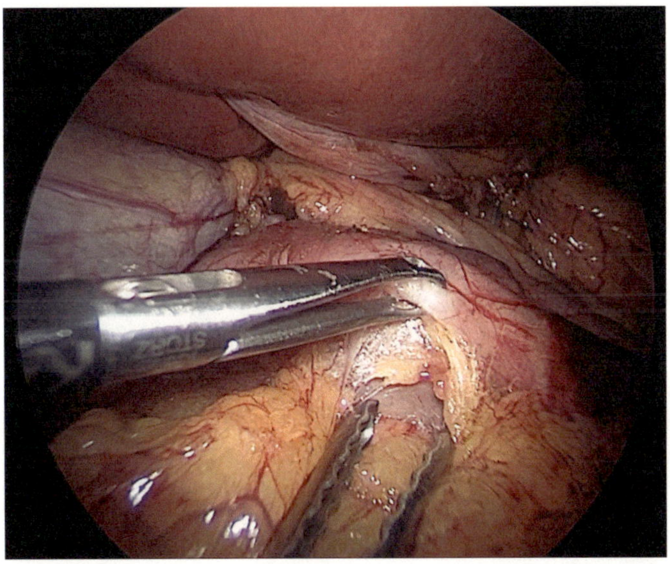

Figure 17. Retroduodenal tunnel.

3.1.4.5. Duodenojejunostomy

The ligament of Treitz is identified as it exits at the root of the transverse mesocolon. A length of jejunum is measured for 200–300 cm starting from the ligament of Treitz. The loop of jejunum is pulled up and a stay suture is placed between the loop of jejunum and pylorus. An enterotomy of 1.5 cm is placed obliquely in the first part of the duodenum and antimesenteric

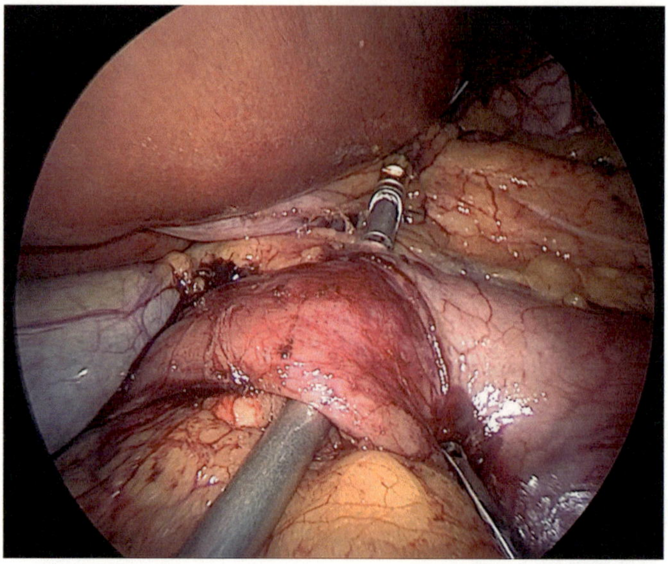

Figure 18. Retroduodenal tunnel passing through the lesser sac using the Goldfinger retractor.

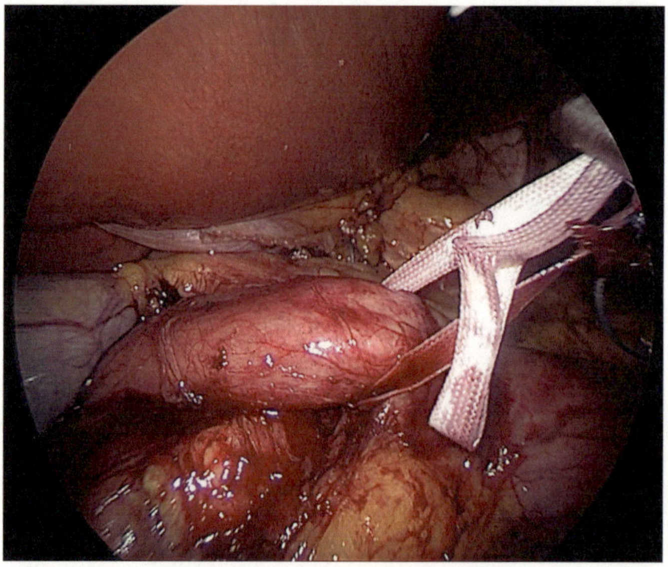

Figure 19. Lifting and retraction of the 1st portion of the duodenum using a tape.

side of jejunum (**Figure 21** and **22**). A completely hand-sewn side to side duodenojejunal anastomosis in a running fashion is created using a 3-0 absorbable glyconate monofilament suture (3-0 B | BRAUN MONOSYN™ UNDYED 28" HR26 TAPER) (**Figures 23–25**). Then an antitorsion suture between antrum and jejunum is placed, around 4 cm proximal to the D-J anastomosis [8].

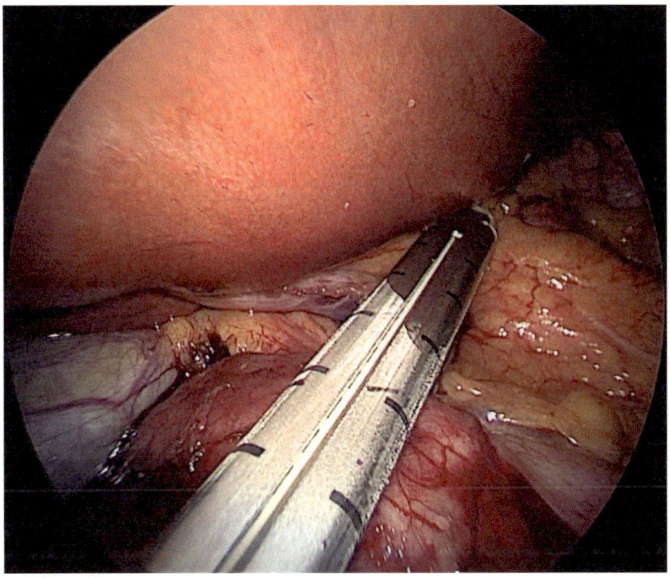

Figure 20. Duodenal transection.

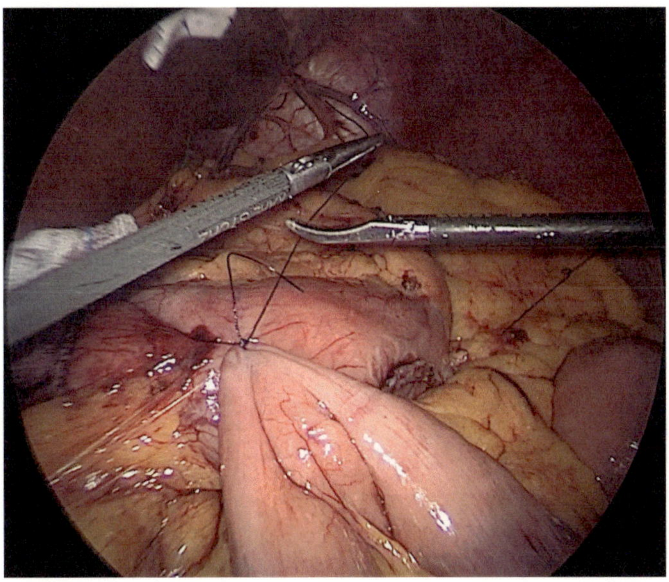

Figure 21. Stay suture between sleeved stomach and jejunum.

3.1.4.6. Closure of mesenteric defect

Peterson's mesenteric defect is closed in a continuous running technique using 2-0 nonabsorbable polyester suture (W6977 Ethibond Excel™ Polyester suture) (**Figure 26**). A Jackson Pratt drain is placed under the entire length of stomach tube and duodenojejunal anastomosis (**Figure 27**).

http://dx.doi.org/10.5772/107288

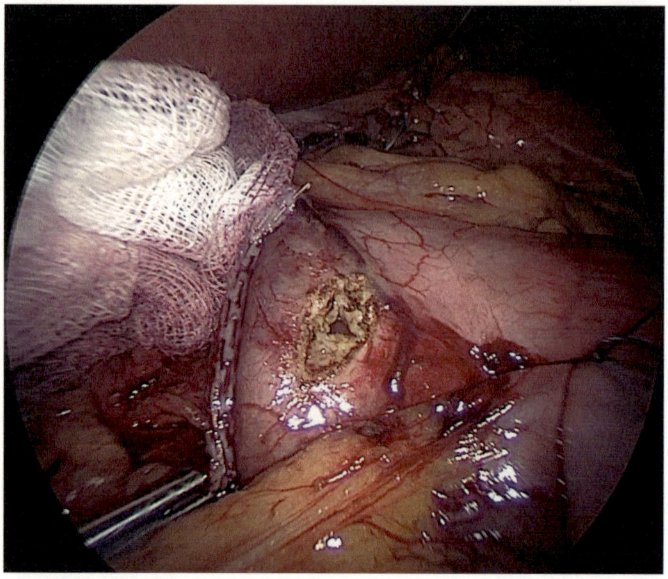

Figure 22. Duodenal enterotomy placed obliquely.

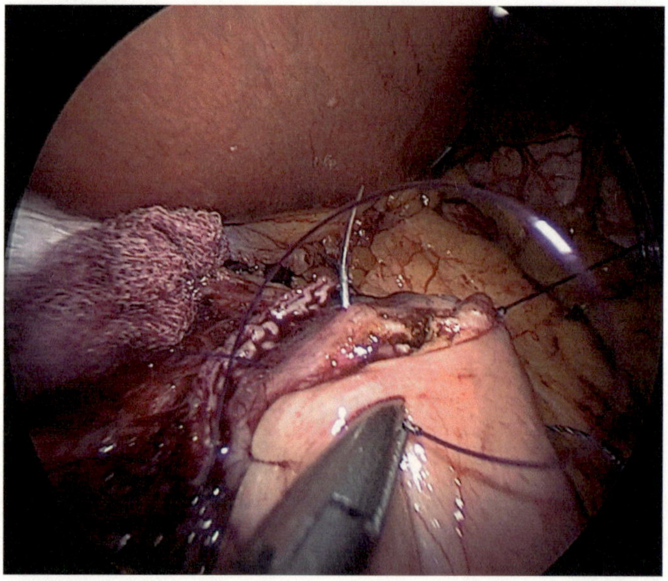

Figure 23. Completely hand-sewn duodenojejunal bypass.

3.1.4.7. Postoperative care and follow-up

Adhering to the early recovery after surgery (ERAS) postoperative protocol, adequate pain control is administered via the intravenous route and early ambulation is encouraged in our patients as early as six hours after surgery in order to avoid pulmonary complications.

Once the patient is fully awake, clear liquid diet as instructed by our dietitian is commenced. Intravenous antibiotic is administered for one more day. Patients are usually discharged 2–3 days after surgery. Patients are placed on bariatric diet as instructed by the dietitian. Proton pump inhibitors are given for 1 month after surgery. Follow-up schedule is as follows: 1 week, 1, 3, 6 and 12 months after surgery. One year after the surgery, patients are advised to follow-up every 6 months thereafter.

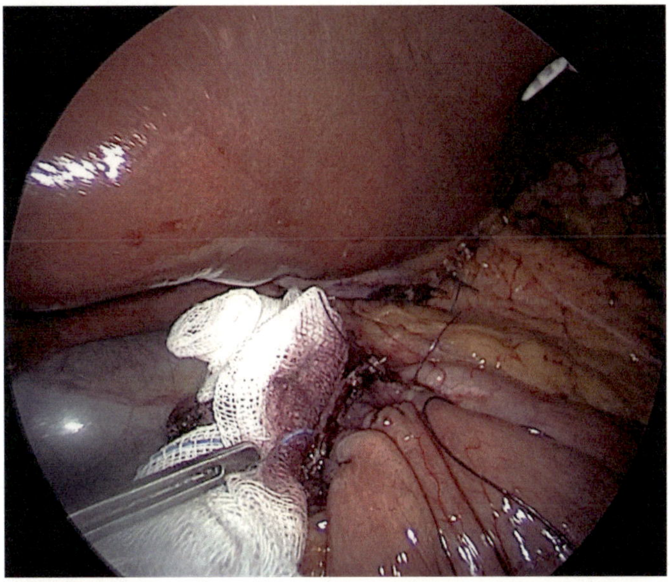

Figure 24. Anterior wall of DJB.

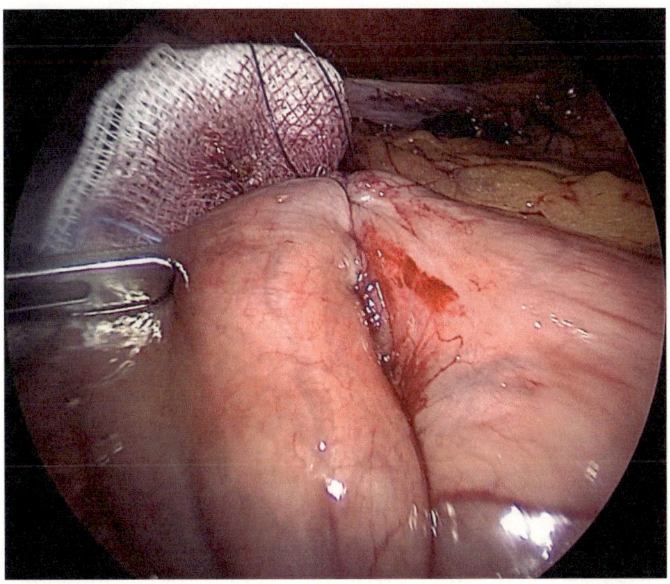

Figure 25. Posterior wall of DJB.

http://dx.doi.org/10.5772/107288

3.1.5. Surgical Outcomes

The mechanism of weight loss in LDJB-SG is due to the resection of Ghrelin-secreting cells located in the fundus of the stomach. A significant drop in this hormone's level after the procedure causes decrease in sensation of hunger and early satiety. Furthermore, aside from its weight-loss effect, caloric restriction also helps in the improvement of insulin resistance and

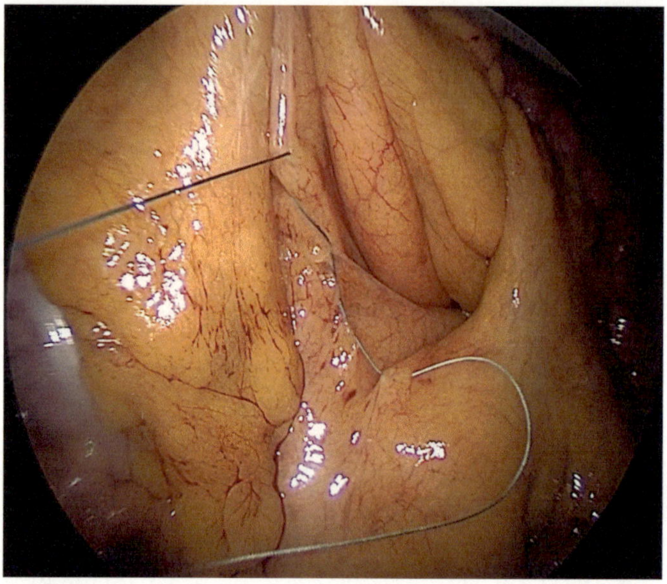

Figure 26. Closure of Petersons defect.

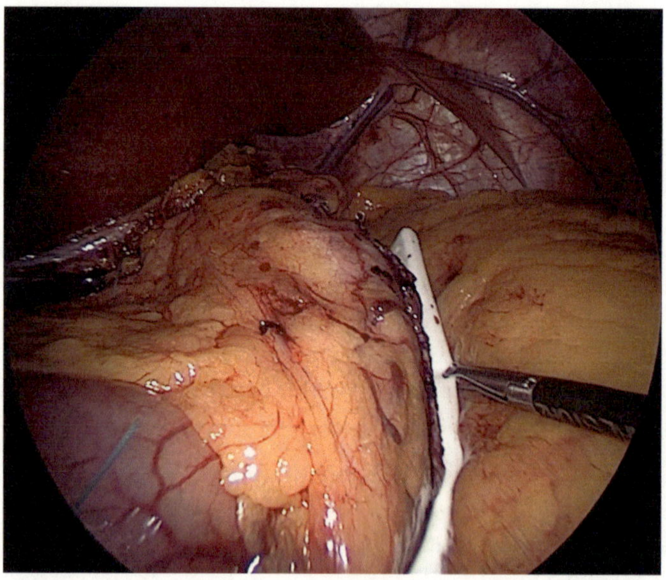

Figure 27. Placement of JP drain along DJB anastomosis and entire length of the sleeve suture line.

increase in glucose tolerance. However, the efficient glycemic control of this procedure is predominantly due to the exclusion of the duodenum (Foregut theory) and the faster delivery of undigested food and more concentrated bile to the distal small bowel (Hindgut theory) which ensures secretion of incretins.

In a prospective study by Huang et al. published in 2013 comparing LDJB-SG with RYGB, LDJB-SG had a superior remission rate of T2DM (60% vs 49%) and a better over-all glycemic control (90% vs 71%) compared to RYGB in patients with BMI ≤ 35 kg/m^2 at 1 year after surgery. Fasting blood sugar levels was also significantly lower in the LDJB-SG group (98.0 ± 18.0 vs 106.0 ± 31.7 mg/dl). The drop in HbA1C was also lower in the LDJB-SG compared to the RYGB (6.0 ± 0.9 vs 6.3 ± 1.2) although this did not attain a statistically significant level (P value = 0.442). Resolution of other obesity-related comorbid factors were also seen in LDJB-SG that was comparable to the RYGB group (Hypertension = 85.7% vs 88.2% and Dyslipidemia = 70% vs 76.6% resolution rates) [8].

In a case-matched study comparing of 30 patients undergoing LDJB-SG and 30 patients undergoing RYGB, the mean BMIs dropped significantly to 22.4 kg/m^2 (±2.4) (range 18.4–27 kg/m^2) and 21.9 kg/m^2 (±2.5) (range 17.7–26.5 kg/m^2) from preoperative values of 28.2 kg/m^2 (±3.6) and 27.8 kg/m^2 (±3.8) at 1 year after surgery ($p < 0.01$). However, no statistical difference was seen between the two groups. HbA1c and fasting glucose were also significantly decreased 1 year after surgery compared to its preoperative value from 8.98 (±1.75%) to 6.52% (±1.03) and 168.3 (±54.9 mg/dL) to 106.5 mg/dL (±28.2 mg/dL). Comparing complete remission of T2DM in 1 year after surgery, the LDJB-SG had a remission rate of 36.6% of patients (11/30) compared to 30% (9/30) in the RYGB group. As far as complications, the rate for early complication favors that of RYGB (1 case vs 4 cases). However, there is a note of a trend toward lower occurrence of late complication rate in LDJB-SG compared to RYGB (5 vs 8 cases, $p < 0.08$) [11].

Lee et al. compared single anastomosis duodenojejunal bypass with sleeve gastrectomy (SADJB-SG) with RYGB and minigastric bypass (MGB). The operation time was significantly longer in SADJB-SG compared to the other types of bypass (181.7 mins vs 160 mins for RYGB vs 120.1 mins for MGB; $p < 0.01$). During the interim follow up period at 1, 3, 6 and 12 months after surgery, the mean BMI dropped to 32.9 ± 4.8, 29.9 ± 6.8, 27.6 ± 5.4 and 25.9 ± 4.6 kg/m^2, respectively. The percentage weight loss during these same follow-up periods were 15.1, 20.3 25 and 32.7%. 12 months after surgery, comparing percent weight loss (% WL) of the three procedures, the results showed a higher percent weight loss for SADJB-SG (32.7 ± 7.9% SADJB-SG vs 28.9 ± 9.0% MGB vs 26.1 ± 4.1% RYGB). Results also showed a superior percent excess weight loss for SADJB-SG (80.3 ± 24.8%) compared to the two bypass procedures (68.6 ± 58.2% MGB and 63.4 ± 31.8% RYGB). In the same report, T2DM was seen in > 80% of the subjects with a preoperative mean HbA1c level of 9.2%. This value decreased to 6.1% 1 year after surgery with a complete remission rate of T2DM in 64% of the patients [12].

In an attempt to evaluate the role of duodenal exclusion in glycemic control, a matched group study comparing LDJB-SG and SG alone was done. At 1 year after surgery, the LDJB-SG (26 patients) presented with a higher percent excess weight loss (87.2 ± 14.9% vs 67 ± 27.0%; $p = 0.23$) and a lower BMI (23.9 ± 2.2 vs 26.1 ± 3.7; $p = 0.065$) compared to the SG

alone group (29 patients). As far as T2DM remission rate is concerned, the LDJB-SG had a 92.3% total glycemic control rate compared to 86.2% in the SG alone group. The mean reduction in the HbA1c level for the LDJB-SG was likewise higher compared to the SG group (2.8 vs 2.1% p = 0.45) [13].

3.2. Sleeve gastrectomy with proximal jejunal bypass (Figure 28)

3.2.1. Indication and contraindication

The indications and contraindications of PJB-SG are the same as that of the conventional stand-alone sleeve gastrectomy. Furthermore, this can also be offered as a metabolic surgery for patients with BMI between 27.5 and 35 with type 2 Diabets.

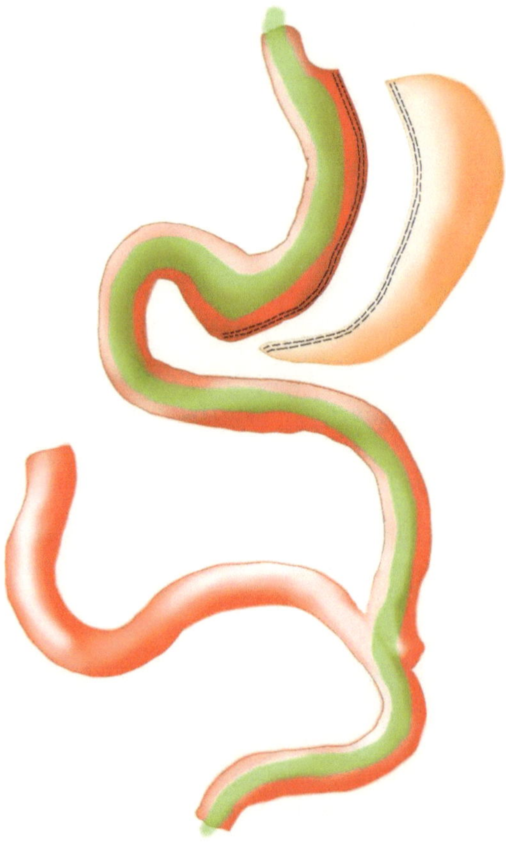

Figure 28. Schematic diagram of LPJB-SG.

3.2.2. Preoperative workup and preparation

Like in all bariatric procedures, a complete preoperative workup should be done in order to select appropriate candidates for the procedure. All patients are evaluated by a multidisciplinary

team dedicated in bariatric surgery including a bariatric surgeon, bariatric physician, gastroenterologist, anesthesiologist, psychiatrist, nutritionist and fitness coach. Other specialists may be called upon if required.

3.2.3. Positioning

Patient is positioned supine with upper extremities abducted and lower extremities adducted. Patient is then secured to the operating table using straps and foot boards. Patient is placed in steep reverse Trendelenburg position.

3.2.4. Operative technique

3.2.4.1. Port placement

A 4-port technique is utilized with the surgeon positioned on the patient's right side and the assistant and camera man standing on the patient's left. Port placement is similar to LSG with an assistant port in left anterior axillary line below the costal margin (**Figure 29**).

3.2.4.2. Pneumoperitoneum

Pneumoperitoneum is accomplished either via Veress technique or through a 12 mm optical trocar using a 30-degree scope in the left periumbilical area.

3.2.4.3. Placement of liver suspension tape

Liver retraction is done using the LST similarly placed as in the standard LSG technique. Alternatively, a Nathanson liver retractor can also be used.

3.2.4.4. Sleeve gastrectomy

Standard sleeve gastrectomy is performed as previously described earlier in this chapter.

3.2.4.5. Proximal jejunal bypass

After completing the sleeve gastrectomy, ligament of Treitz is identified. Transection of the jejunum is done at 20 cm from the ligament of Treitz using either a 45 mm white cartridge reload (EGIA45AMT Endo GIA™ 45 mm articulating medium/thick reload with Tri-Staple Technology) or a 45 mm white cartridge reload (ECR45W Echelon Endopath™ tri-stapler reload cartridges by Ethicon). Next 300 cm of small bowel is measured distally and a side-to-side jejunojejunal anastomosis was fashioned out using the same cartridge and stapling device. The jejunojejunostomy is created with hand-sewn technique using 3-0 Absorbable Glyconate Monofilament running suture (3-0 B | BRAUN MONOSYN™ UNDYED 28" HR26 TAPER) (**Figures 30–32**).

3.2.4.6. Closure of mesenteric defect

The mesenteric defect is closed with simple running sutures using 2-0 nonabsorbable polyester suture (Ethibond Excel™ polyester suture). No drain is placed.

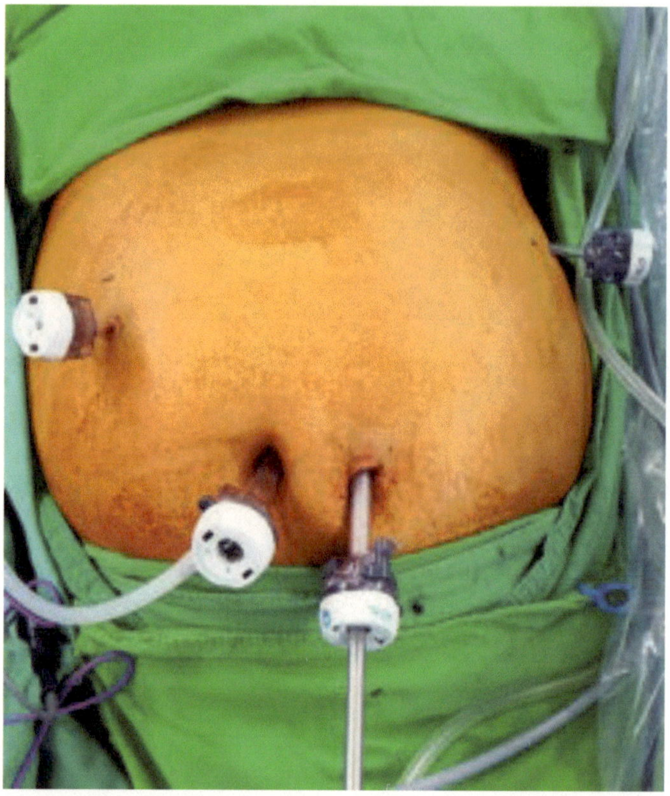

Figure 29. LPJB-SG port placement.

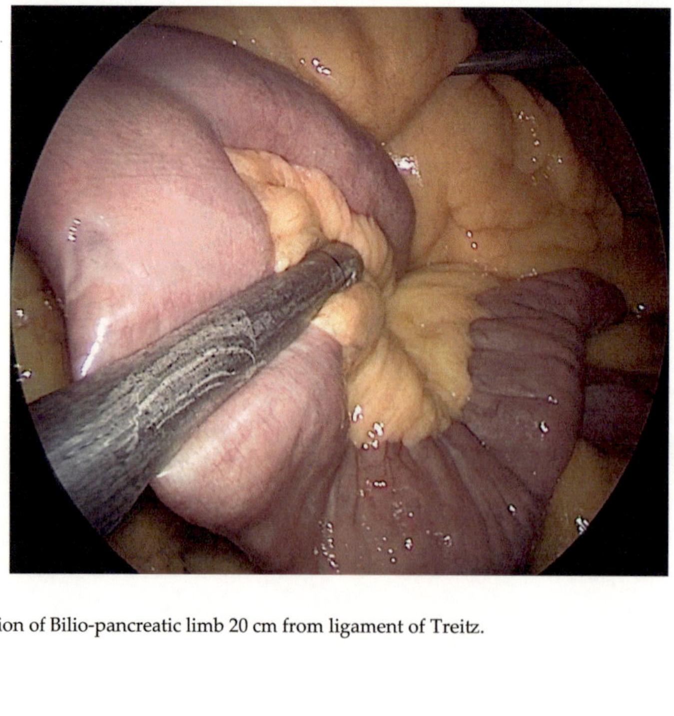

Figure 30. Transection of Bilio-pancreatic limb 20 cm from ligament of Treitz.

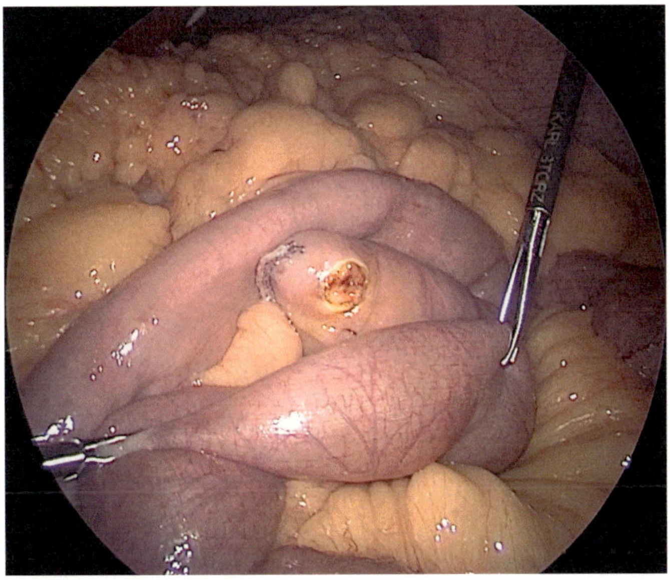

Figure 31. 300 cm bypassed proximal jejunum.

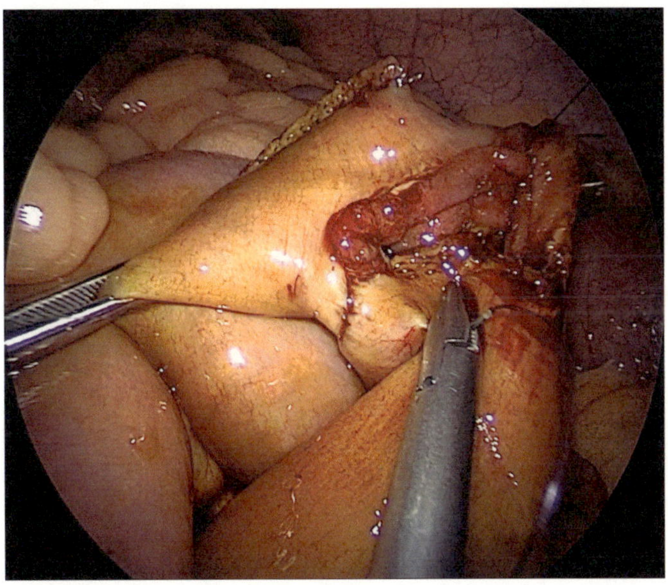

Figure 32. Closure of jejunojejunal anastomosis.

3.2.4.7. Gastric sleeve fixation

The suture line of the sleeved stomach is anchored with one or two stitches at the retroperitoneal fat using 3-0 Polyglactin 910 multifilament absorbable suture (J774D Ethicon 3-0 Coated Vicryl™ Taper SH). This prevents inadvertent twisting of the tubularized stomach (**Figure 33**).

http://dx.doi.org/10.5772/107288

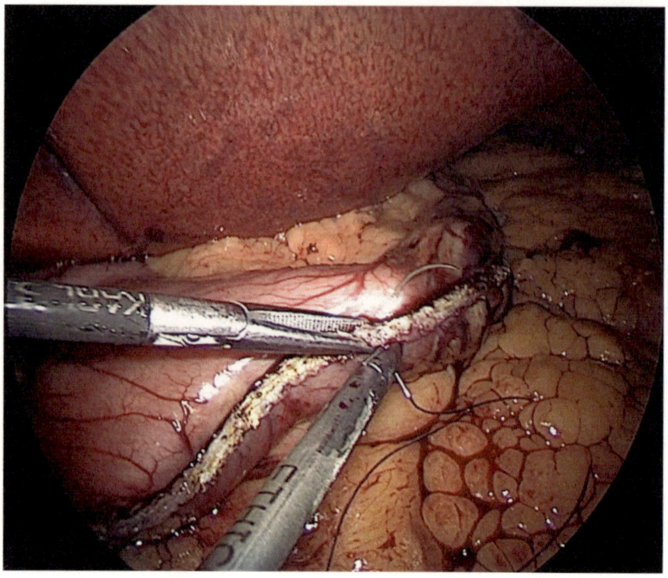

Figure 33. Anti torsion stitch.

3.2.5. Surgical Outcomes

Factors that contribute to the magnitude of weight loss and diabetic remission in sleeve-based procedures are still not fully elucidated. It probably owes its weight loss capabilities by eliminating the function of the stomach as a reservoir hereby reducing caloric content of processed food. Furthermore, because of the jejunojejunal bypass, the terminal ileum is exposed much earlier to undigested food and a more concentrated bile, both of which stimulate the release of incretins, primarily glucagon-like peptide 1 (GLP-1).

In the original study of Alamo et al., the average BMI and average weight at 12 months after vertical isolated gastroplasty with gastroenteral bypass were 23.4 ± 3.3 kg/m^2 (19.2–27.7) and 65.1 ± 15 kg (46–83) from 41.2 ± 5.1 kg/m^2 (35.3–57.8) and 110.7 ± 16.2 kg. The mean percent excess weight loss (% EWL) was 90.2 ± 11.9% [3]. In other studies, the mean BMI was reduced to 21.4 ± 1.9 kg/m^2 at 18 months' follow-up from 31.6 ± 2.1 kg/m^2 with a mean percent EWL of 75.7 ± 8.5%. Comparing these figures with RYGB, in the study by Higa et al., where patients were followed-up for 10 years, the mean percent excess weight loss was 57% and the average postoperative BMI was 33 ± 8.0 kg/m^2 at 10 years [14].

In a cohort study of 49 patients (2012) evaluating the efficacy of SGPJB in ameliorating T2DM in patients with BMI < 35 kg/m^2, 81.6% (40/48) of patients with T2DM achieved complete remission after SGPJB with the remaining nine patients achieving improvement. As far as discontinuation of oral hyperglycemic agents and insulin dependence are concerned, 97.6% (40/41) of patients stopped taking their medications and 100% (8/8) stopped using insulin [10].

4. Laparoscopic Roux-En-Y Gastric Bypass (Figure 34)

Mason observed that distal gastrectomy with Billroth II reconstruction causes weight loss. The first open RYGB was performed for weight loss in 1967 while the first Laparoscopic RYGB was performed by Wittgrove [15]. Since then, laparoscopic RYGB is one of the most commonly performed bariatric procedure done for excess weight loss (**Figure 34**).

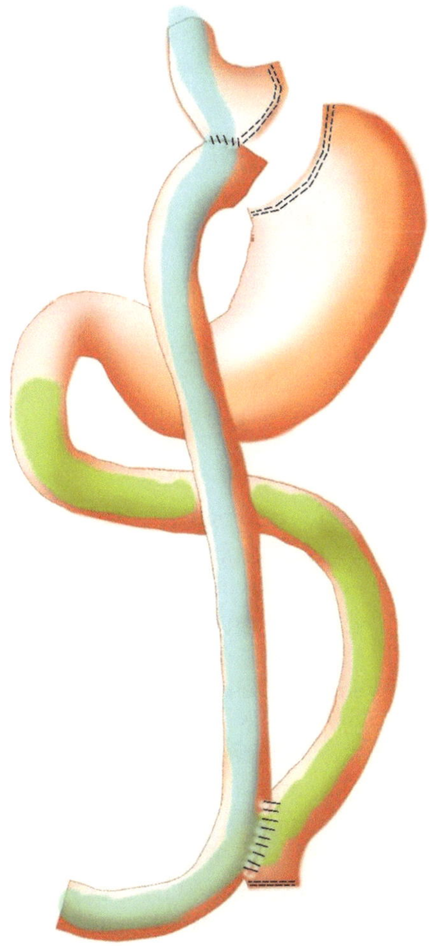

Figure 34. Schematic diagram of LRYGB.

Based on the 1991 NIH criteria, there are a number of widely accepted indication and contraindication which make a patient suitable for Bariatric or weight loss surgery:

- BMI > 40 without comorbidities.
- >35 with associated obesity-related illness such as diabetes or sleep apnea.
- Failed reasonable attempts at other weight loss techniques.

- Obesity-related health problems.
- No psychiatric or drug dependency problems.
- A capacity to understand the risks and commitment associated with surgery.
- Pregnancy not anticipated in the first 2 years following surgery.

For Asians, BMI is reduced by 2.5 for the above.

4.1. Operative technique

4.1.1. General preparations

Preoperative investigation includes standard basic blood profile, thyroid function test, serum cortisol level, HbA1c and C-peptide if diabetic, whole abdominal ultrasound and upper gastrointestinal endoscopy. Patient will be placed on NPO and started with intravenous drip 125–150 ml/h. Anticoagulants are usually not needed but thromboelastic stockings are applied.

4.1.2. Patient positioning

Patient is positioned supine with both arms stretched out. Surgeon will be on the right side of the patient while the assistant surgeon and camera holder will be on the left. The assisting nurse will stand on the same side as the surgeon. Monitor(s) are placed at the head end of patient.

4.1.3. Port placement

A 12 mm optical port placed 3-finger breadth left lateral to umbilicus. A 5 mm port is placed 4-finger breadth to the right of umbilicus for surgeons left hand working port. A 12 mm port is placed at 45 degrees to right hand port in the right mid clavicular line for surgeon's left hand and stapler insertion. Another 5 mm port is inserted in upper left subcostal region in the anterior axillary line for assistant surgeon (**Figure 35**).

4.1.4. Liver suspension tape

Liver retraction is done with liver suspension tape using a straight needle prolene suture-Jackson Pratt drain as previously described in this chapter for LSG.

4.1.5. Creation of gastric pouch

Gastric pouch is created by marking with orogastric calibration tube (OGCT) balloon with 25 ml insufflation. Perigastric dissection is done with hook diathermy at lesser curve with preservation of hepatic branch of vagus nerve, usually after the first vascular branch. Two-three staplers (medium thickness) are used to create the gastric pouch. The final pouch size would be about 15–20 ml. Adhesion on the posterior aspect of gastric pouch are cleared. A small gastrostomy is created at the posterior side of the pouch with hook diathermy for the creation of gastrojejunostomy (**Figures 36–42**).

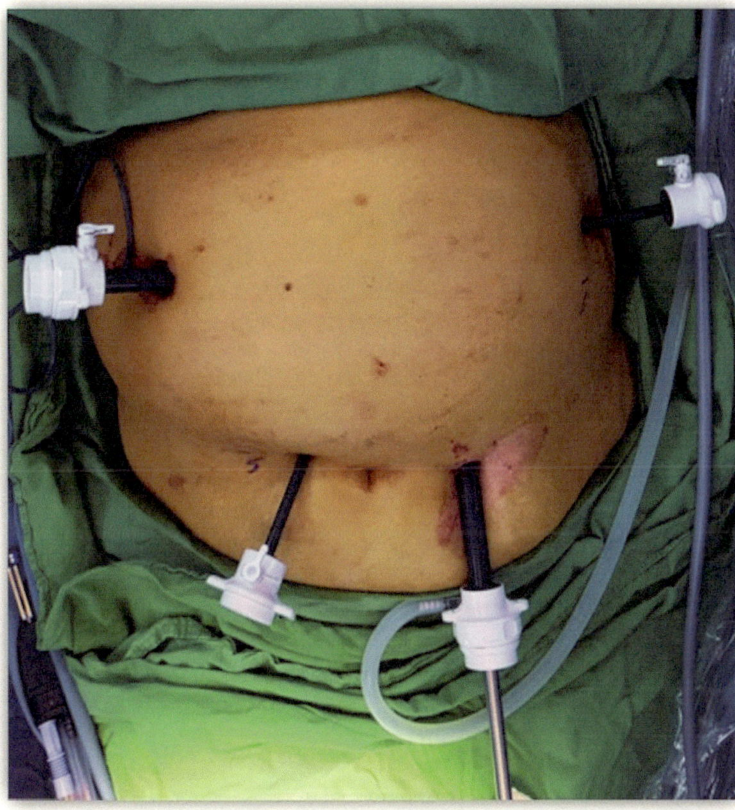

Figure 35. Port placement.

4.1.6. Gastrojejunostomy

Ligament of Treitz is identified and 100 cm of proximal jejunum is measured. Jejunotomy is created with hook cautery and loop of jejunum is anastomosed to the gastric pouch with linear stapler. Diameter of the gastrojejunal stoma is about 1.5–2 cm. Jejunum is disconnected just proximal to gastrojejunostomy with a 45 mm white cartridge reload (EGIA45AMT Endo GIA™ 45 mm articulating thin reload with Tri-Staple Technology or ECR45W Echelon Endopath™ tri-stapler reload cartridges by Ethicon) to avoid creating a "candy cane" blind loop. Closure of gastrojejunal enterotomy is performed with Monocryl 3-0. 38 Fr orogastric tube is passed through the gastrojejunal anastomosis to check for patency (**Figures 43–46**).

4.1.7. Jejunojejunostomy

Jejunum is measured for a distance of 100 cm from gastrojejunostomy and side to side jejunojejunostomy is created with 45 mm cartridge (EGIA45AMT Endo GIA™ 45 mm articulating thin reload with Tri-Staple Technology or ECR45W Echelon Endopath™ tri-stapler reload cartridges by Ethicon). Closure of jejunojejunal enterotomy is done with 3-0 Monocryl (**Figures 47** and **48**).

http://dx.doi.org/10.5772/107288

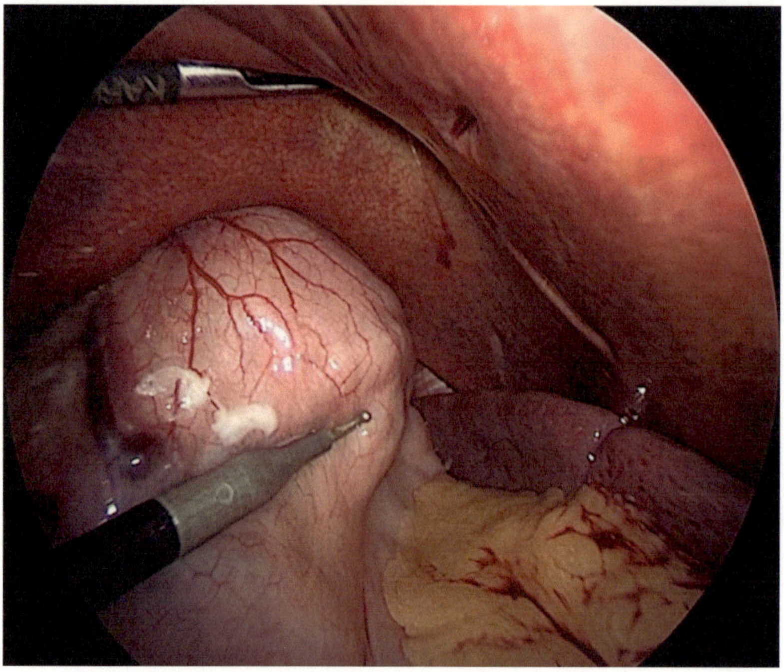

Figure 36. Calibration of gastric pouch.

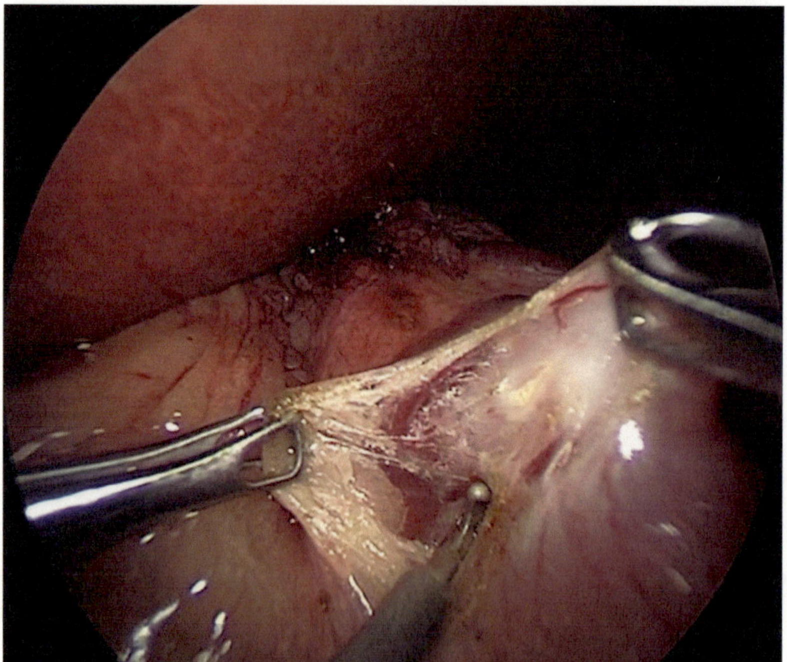

Figure 37. Perigastric dissection.

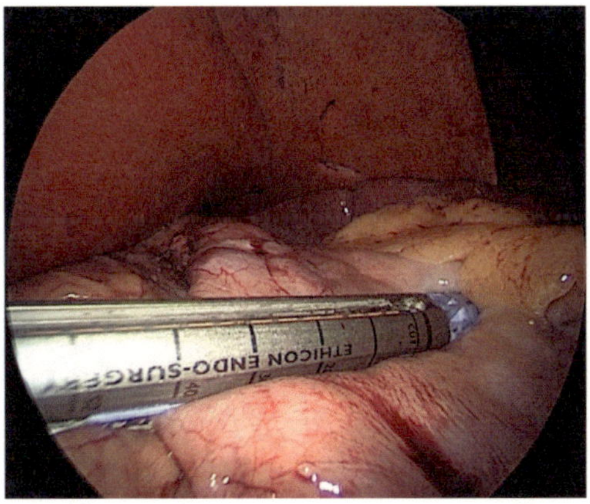

Figure 38. Firing of first staple.

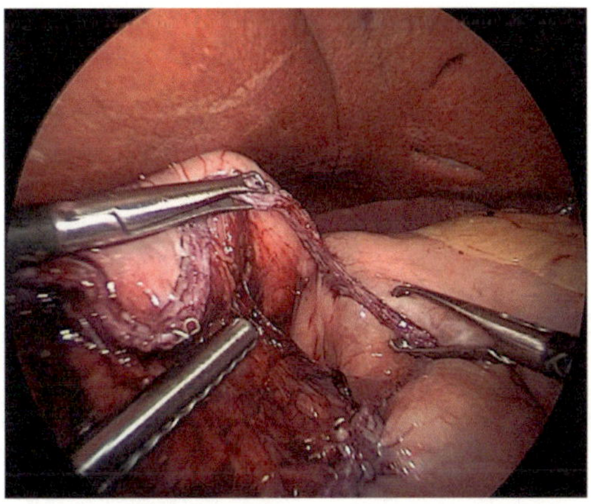

Figure 39. Dissection of adhesions at posterior gastric pouch.

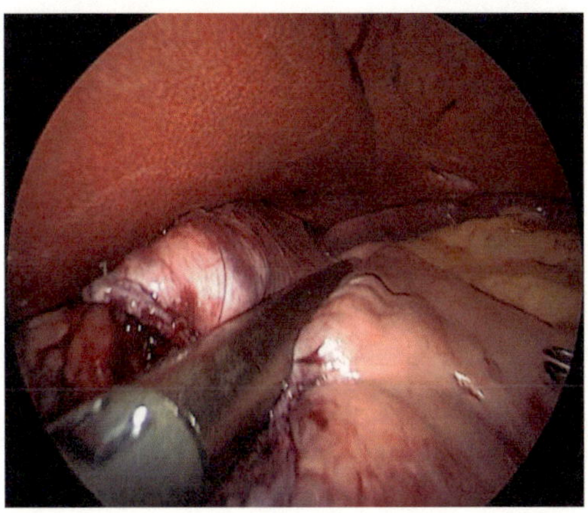

Figure 40. Firing of the 2nd stapler toward the angle of His.

http://dx.doi.org/10.5772/107288

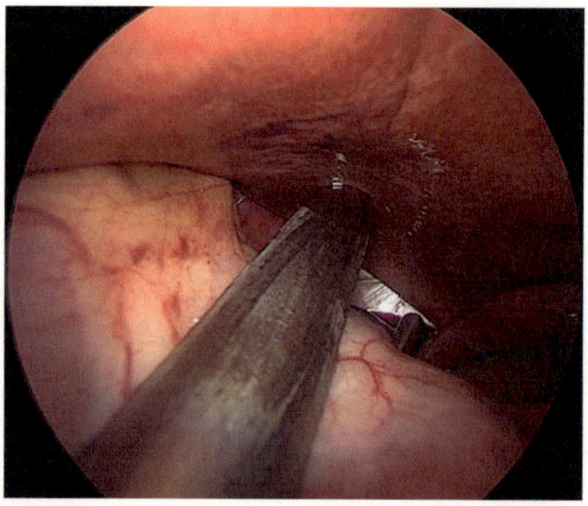

Figure 41. Firing of last stapler 1 cm away from GE junction.

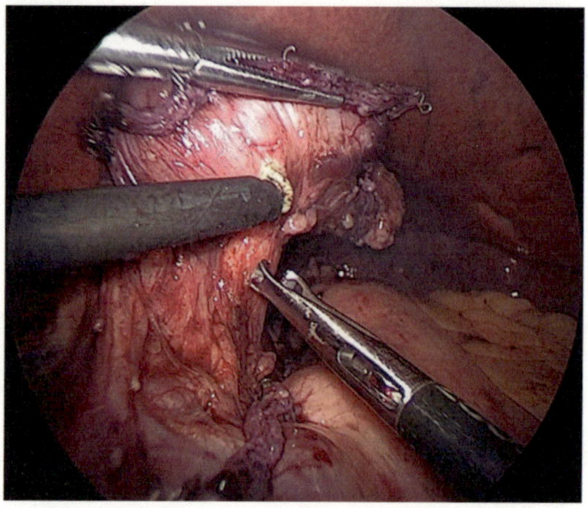

Figure 42. Creation of 1.5–2 cm gastrotomy.

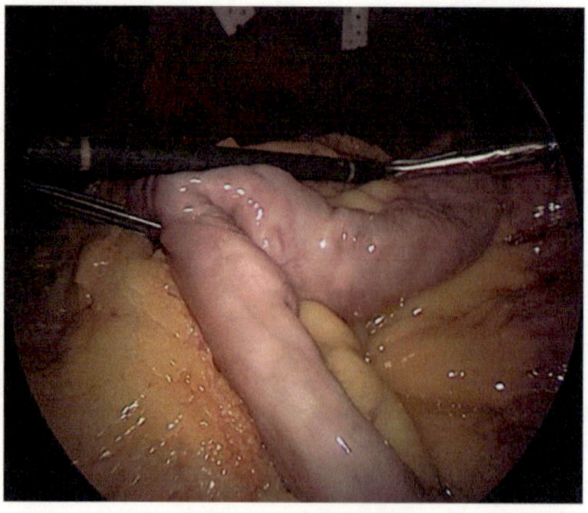

Figure 43. BP limb measuring 100–250 cm from the ligament of Treitz.

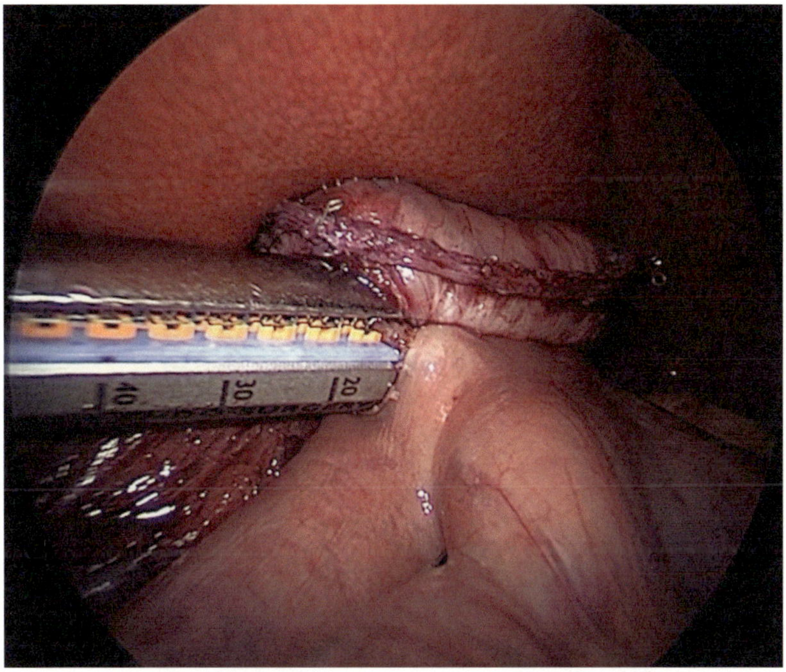

Figure 44. 1.5–2 cm side to side gastrojejunostomy.

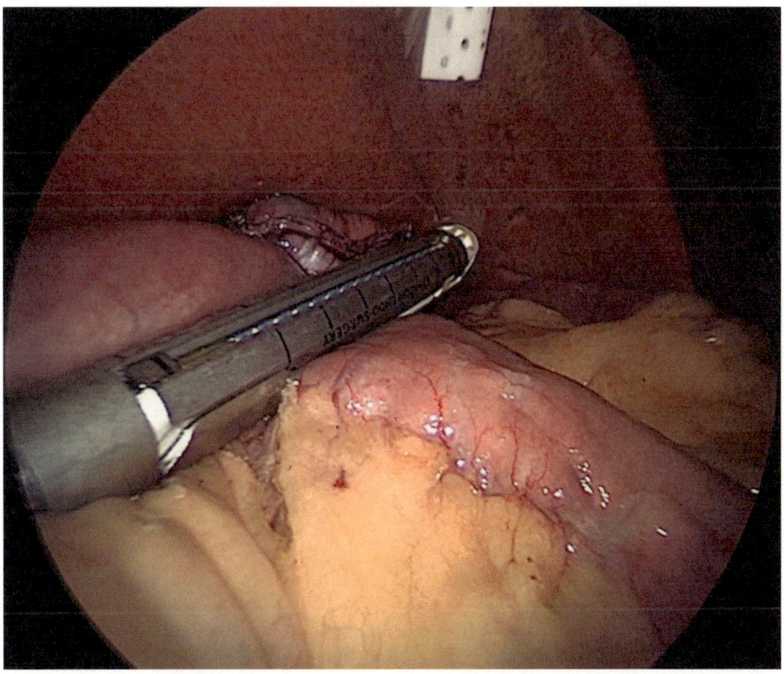

Figure 45. Transection of jejunum proximal to GJ anastomosis with thin stapler as close to GJ anastomosis as possible to avoid creating a candy cane stick blind loop.

http://dx.doi.org/10.5772/107288

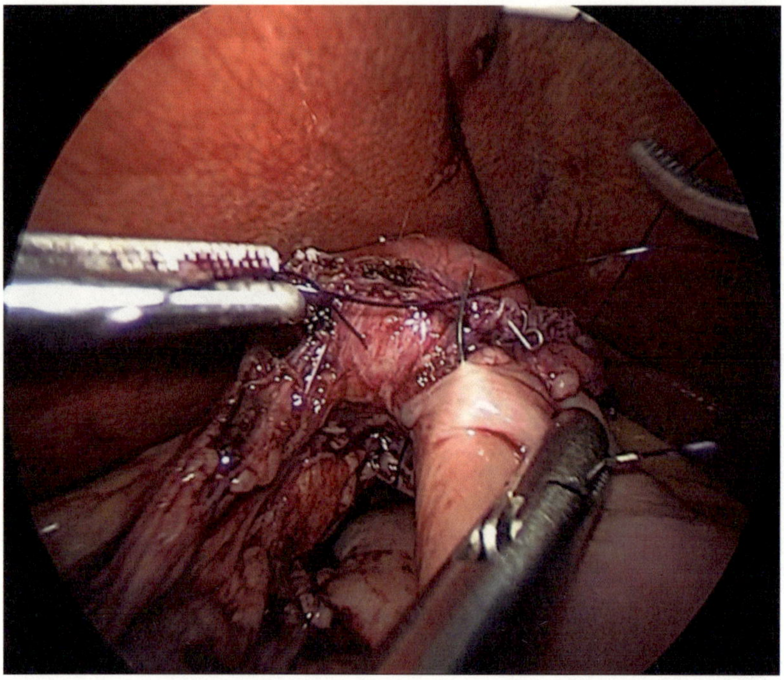

Figure 46. Gastrojejunal anastomosis completed by closure with single layer continuous suture using MONOSYN 3-0 round body needle.

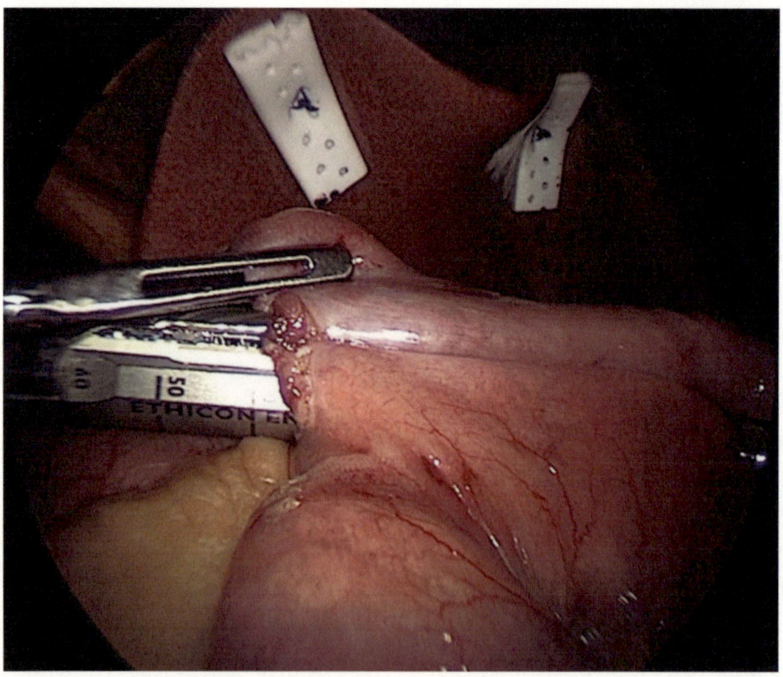

Figure 47. Side to side jejunojejunostomy.

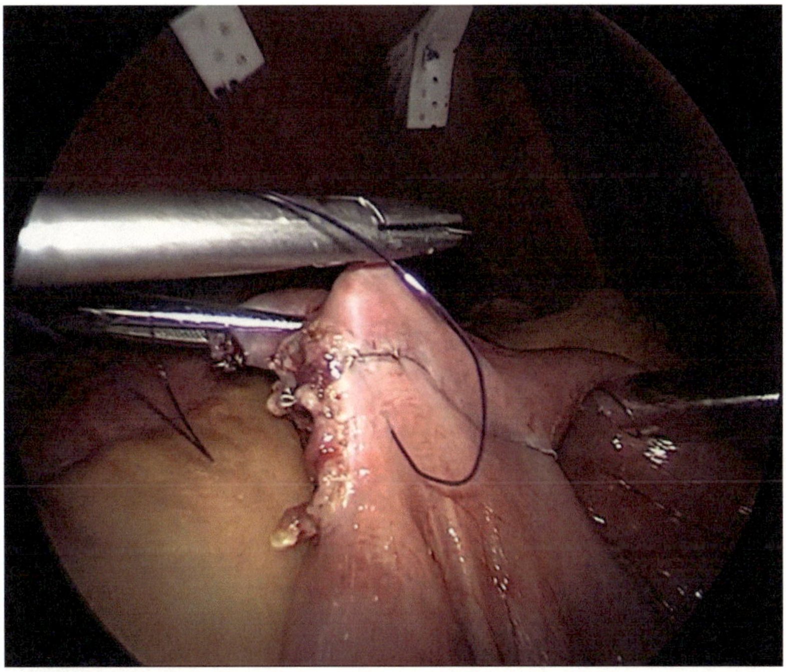

Figure 48. Hand-sewn closure of jejunojejunal anastomosis completed with single layer continuous suture using MONOSYN 3-0 round body needle.

4.1.8. Closure of mesenteric defects

Closure of mesenteric defects is performed with nonabsorbable sutures at jejunojejunal mesentery and Peterson defect (jejunotransverse mesocolon) to prevent internal herniation.

4.1.9. Removal of liver suspension, hemostasis, deflation and closure

After ensuring hemostasis at staple lines and anastomosis, liver suspension tapes are removed and hemostasis of liver punctures is done with diathermy.

4.2. Surgical outcome

4.2.1. Excess weight loss

Weight loss after bariatric surgery is dramatically seen in the first 12 months after surgery and continues at a slower rate up to 18 months postoperation. Excess weight loss after gastric bypass is between 72 and 82% within 12 months after surgery [16–18].

4.2.2. Improvement of comorbidities

Gastric bypass resulted in marked improvement in the biochemical markers of diabetes. Type 2 Diabetes Mellitus resolution is as high as 90.9% with mean fasting glucose reduction from 204 to 103 mg/dl, mean HbA1c reduction from 9.2 to 5.9% without T2DM medication in 12 months follow up. Up to 90% of patient did not need medication for control of glycaemia post operatively [19].

Gastric bypass can achieve a dramatic improvement of nonalcoholic fatty liver disease (NAFLD) both biochemically and histologically in morbid obesity [20]. Likewise, with significant weight loss and reduction of BMI after gastric bypass, pulmonary function improved in obese patients, which are correlated with decrease in waist circumference and possibly intra-abdominal pressure [21].

4.2.3. *Complications*

Complications occur in up to 20% patients and include anastomotic leak (0.25%), acute and late gastrojejuntostomy stricture (5%), gastrojejunostomy hemorrhage (1.5%), acute and late jejunojejunostomy stricture (1.5%), iron deficiency anemia, marginal ulcers hemorrhage (1.5%), gastric pouch dilatation (1.5%), nonspecific abdominal pain, hair loss, internal herniation if mesenteric defects are not closed and rarely peroneal nerve palsy, acute cholecystitis, biliary stone with obstruction and cholangitis and intra-abdominal abscess [16–18].

Author details

Chih Kun Huang[1*], Sir Emmanuel S. Astudillo[2], Prasad M. Bhukebag[1] and Khan Wei Chan[1]

*Address all correspondence to: dr.ckhuang@hotmail.com

1 Body Science and Metabolic Disorders International (B.M.I.) Medical Center, China Medical University Hospital, Taichung City, Taiwan

2 Center for Diabetes, Nutrition & Weight Management, The Medical City Clark, Pampanga, Philippines

References

[1] Buchwald H, Avidor Y, Braunwald E, Jensen MD, Pories W, Fahrbach K, Schoelles K. Bariatric surgery: a systematic review and meta-analysis. JAMA. 2004;292(14):1724–1737.

[2] Rubino F, Nathan DM, Eckel RH, Schauer PR, Alberti KG, Zimmet PZ, Del Prato S, Ji L, Sadikot SM, Herman WH, Amiel SA, Kaplan LM, Taroncher-Oldenburg G, Cummings DE. Metabolic surgery in the treatment algorithm for type 2 diabetes: a joint statement by international diabetes organizations. Dia Care. 2016;39.6: 861–877. Web.

[3] Langer FB, Reza Hoda MA, Bohdjalian A, Felberbauer FX, Zacherl J, Wenzi E, Schindler K, Luger A, Ludvik B, Pregaer G. Sleeve gastrectomy and gastric banding: effects on plasma ghrelin levels. Obes Surg 2005;15(70):1024–1029.

[4] Himpens J, Dobbeleir J, Peeters G. Long-term results of laparoscopic sleeve gastrectomy for obesity. Ann Surg 2010;252 (2):319–324.

[5] Basso N, Leonetti F, Mariani P, et al. Early hormonal changes after sleeve gastrectomy in diabetic obese patients. Obes Surg. 2010;20(1):50–55.

[6] Arman GA, Himpens J, Dhaenens J, et al. Long-term (11+years) outcomes in weight, patient satisfaction, comorbidities, and gastroesophageal reflux treatment after laparoscopic sleeve gastrectomy. Surg Obes Relat Dis 2016. [Epub ahead of print]. 10.1016/j.soard.2016.01.013

[7] Huang CK, Goel R, Tai CM, et al. Novel metabolic surgery for type 2 diabetes mellitus: loop duodenojejunal bypass with sleeve gastrectomy. Surg Laparosc Endosc Percutan Tech 2013 Dec;23(6):481–485.

[8] Huang CK, Ahluwalia JS, Garg A, Taweerutchana V, Ooi A, Chang PC, Hsin MC, et al. Novel Metabolic/Bariatric Surgery—Loop Duodenojejunal Bypass with Sleeve Gastrectomy (LDJB-SG). Essential and Controversies in Bariatric Surgery. 2014 Chapter 7: 133–144.

[9] Alamo MA, Torres CS, Perez LZ, et al. Vertical isolated gastroplasty with gastro-enteral bypass: preliminary results. Obes Surg. 2006;16:353–358.

[10] Alamo M, Sepulveda M, Gellona J, Herrera M, Astorga C, Manterola C, et al. Sleeve gastrectomy with jejunal bypass for the treatment of type 2 diabetes mellitus in patients with body mass index <35 kg/m^2: a cohort study. Obes Surg. 2012;22:1097–1103.

[11] Huang CK, Tai CM, Chang PC, Malapan K, Tsai CC, Yolsuriyanwong K et al. Loop duodenojejunal bypass with sleeve gastrectomy: comparative study with Roux-en-Y gastric bypass in type 2 diabetic patients with a BMI <35 kg/m^2, first year results. Obes Surg. 2016;26(10):1–11.

[12] Lee WJ, Lee KT, Kasama K, Seike Y, Ser KH, Chun SC, Chen JC, Lee YC, et al. Laparoscopic single-anastomosis duodenal–jejunal bypass with sleeve gastrectomy (SADJB-SG): short-term result and comparison with gastric bypass. Obes Surg. 2014;24:109–113.

[13] Lee WJ, Almulai AM, Tsou JJ, Ser KH, Lee YC, Chen SC, et al. Duodenal–jejunal bypass with sleeve gastrectomy versus the sleeve gastrectomy procedure alone: the role of duodenal exclusion. Surg Obes Relat Dis. 2015 Jul–Aug; 11(4):765–770.

[14] Higa K, Ho T, Tercero F, Yunus, T, Boone K, et al. Laparoscopic Roux-en-Y gastric bypass: 10-year follow-up. Surg Obes Relat Dis. 2011;7:516–525.

[15] Wittgrove, et al. Laparoscopic gastric bypass, Roux-en-Y: preliminary report of 5 cases. Obes Surg. 1994;4:353–357.

[16] Huang, et al. Laparoscopic Roux-en-Y gastric bypass for morbidly obese Chinese patients: learning curve, advocacy and complications. Obes J. 2008; 18:776–781.

[17] Huang, et al. Use of individual surgeon versus surgical team approach: surgical team outcomes of laparoscopic Roux-en-Y gastric bypass in an Asian medical center. Surg Obes Relat Dis. 2012;8:214–219.

[18] Sjostrom L. Review of the key results from the Swedish obese subjects (SOS) trial—a prospective controlled intervention study of bariatric surgery. J Inter Med. 2013; 273(3):219–34.

http://dx.doi.org/10.5772/107288

[19] Huang, et al. Laparoscopic Roux-en-Y gastric bypass for the treatment of Type II diabetes mellitus in Chinese patients with body mass index of 25–35. Obes Surg. 2011;21:1344–1349.

[20] Tai et al. Improvement of non-alcoholic fatty liver disease after bariatric surgery in morbidly obese Chinese patients. Obes Surg. 2012;22:1016–1021.

[21] Wei, et al. Surgically induced weight loss, including reduction in waist circumference, is associated with improved pulmonary function in obese patients. Surg Obes Relat Dis. 2011;7:599–604.

Chapter 3

Laparoscopic Pancreas Surgery: Image Guidance Solutions

Juan A. Sánchez-Margallo, Thomas Langø,
Erlend F. Hofstad, Ronald Mårvik and
Francisco M. Sánchez-Margallo

Additional information is available at the end of the chapter

http://dx.doi.org/10.5772/66171

Abstract

Pancreatic ductal adenocarcinoma (PDA) is the fourth leading cause of cancer-related deaths. Surgery is the only viable treatment, but irradical resection rates are still high. Laparoscopic pancreatic surgery has some technical limitations for surgeons and tumor identification may be challenging. Image-guided techniques provide intraoperative margin assessment and visualization methods, which may be advantageous in guiding the surgeon to achieve curative resections and therefore improve the surgical outcomes. In this chapter, current available laparoscopic surgical approaches and image-guided techniques for pancreatic surgery are reviewed. Surgical outcomes of pancreaticoduodenectomy and distal pancreatectomy performed by laparoscopy, laparoendoscopic single-site surgery (LESS), and robotic surgery are included and analyzed. Besides, image-guided techniques such as intraoperative near-infrared fluorescence imaging and surgical navigation are presented as emerging techniques. Results show that minimally invasive procedures reported a reduction of blood loss, reduced length of hospital stay, and positive resection margins, as well as an improvement in spleen-preserving rates, when compared to open surgery. Studies reported that fluorescence-guided pancreatic surgery might be beneficial in cases where the pancreatic anatomy is difficult to identify. The first approach of a surgical navigation system for guidance during pancreatic resection procedures is presented, combining preoperative images (CT and MRI) with intraoperative laparoscopic ultrasound imaging.

Keywords: pancreatic cancer, laparoendoscopic single-site surgery, robotic surgery, image-guided surgery, surgical navigation, near-infrared fluorescence

1. Introduction

Cancer is the second leading cause of death worldwide after heart disease, with 14.9 million cases and 8.2 million deaths in 2013 [1, 2] and the first leading cause of death among adults aged 40–79 years [3, 4]. Worldwide, pancreatic ductal adenocarcinoma (PDA) is the fourth leading cause of cancer-related deaths [2, 3]. The incidence of all types of pancreatic cancer ranges from 1 to 10 cases per 100,000 people and is generally higher in developed countries and among men [1, 2]. This has remained stable for the past 30 years relative to the incidence of other common solid tumors [5]. Each year about 233,000 new cases of pancreatic cancer are diagnosed worldwide [2, 3]. In the United States, the American Cancer Association expected about 48,960 (24,840 men and 24,120 women) cases of incidence in pancreatic cancer in 2015, with a mortality rate of 83% [6]. In Europe, the estimated number of new cases of pancreatic cancer in 2012 was 79,331 and the estimated number of cases of deaths was 78,669 [7, 8], which is almost the double than in the United States. The 5-year survival rate in the world for pancreatic cancer is still very low, with only 6%. In addition, the overall 2-year survival rate is less than 10%, which has hardly improved over the past two decades [3–5]. In fact, in contrast to the stable or declining trends for most cancer types in the United States, a trend analysis for 2001–2010 indicated that death rates are rising for pancreatic cancer [3, 4].

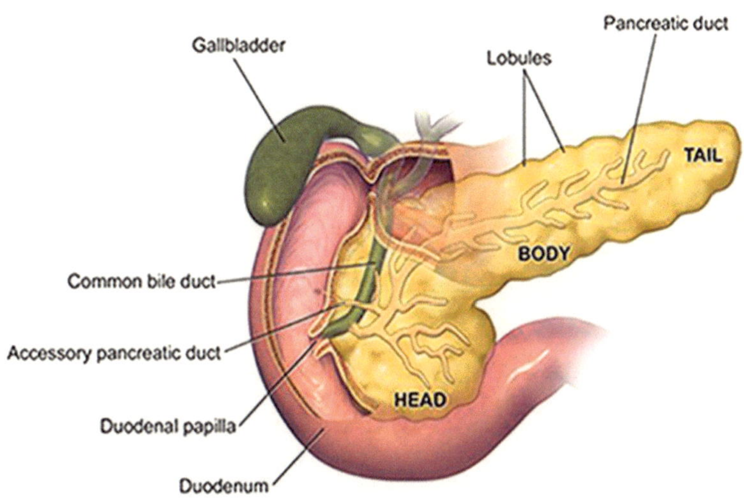

Figure 1. Anatomy of the pancreas. *Source:* "Blausen Gallery 2014". Wikiversity Journal of Medicine. DOI: 10.15347/wjm/2014.010. ISSN 20018762.

Pancreatic tumors are mainly classified as exocrine and endocrine tumors, also known as pancreatic neuroendocrine tumors (NETs). Exocrine tumors are approximately 99% of all primary pancreatic tumors [9] and are divided into ductal adenocarcinomas (80–90% of exocrine tumors), cystic neoplasms, and solid pseudopapillary neoplasms [5, 6, 10]. Ductal adenocarcinomas usually begin in the ducts of the pancreas and are located in the head of the pancreas (60–70%) (**Figure 1**) [10]. Approximately 5–10% of PDA cases are believed to be due

to hereditary conditions, such as hereditary pancreatitis, Gardner syndrome, familial colon cancer, and others [11].

Pancreatic cases are usually diagnosed at an advanced stage but with few treatment options available. This is attributed primarily to a lack of reliable methods for early diagnosis and rapid metastasis of pancreatic cancer [12]. At the time of diagnosis, less than 20% of patients with pancreatic cancer present with localized, potentially curable tumors [13, 14]. Approximately, 30% of patients receive a diagnosis of advanced loco-regional disease. In addition, 30% of patients have local recurrence of tumors after treatment for an early disease [14].

Although there are several available treatments for pancreatic cancer such as ablative techniques, radiation therapies, and chemotherapy, surgery is the only viable treatment. However, only 10–20% of pancreatic tumors are candidates to be surgically resected at diagnosis [10, 15]. The required surgical intervention for pancreatic cancer treatment depends on the location of tumors. Cancers arising in the head of the pancreas require a pancreaticoduodenectomy (Whipple operation), while those in the tail require a distal pancreatectomy with or without splenectomy [16]. Lesions located in the neck and body may require a distal pancreatectomy, pancreaticoduodenectomy or, rarely, a total pancreatectomy. After surgery, patients with no positive resection margins (R0) have the most favorable prognosis [17]. The median survival length reported for resected (R0) pancreatic cancer ranges from 17–27 months and, after a R1 resection, the average survival length is 10.3 months [18]. However, irradical resection of pancreatic cancers still occurs in 35–42% of patients [16, 19]. This survival time is longer in patients with malignant disease localized to the pancreas and less than 3 cm in diameter than in patients with tumors of greater size or with retroperitoneal invasion (6–15 months) [13]. Other factors, such as tumor size, lymph node status, tumor grade and blood vessel invasion, are also correlated with prognosis [20].

The introduction of minimally invasive surgical techniques in the treatment of pancreatic cancer has allowed almost any pancreatic tumor to be operated by laparoscopic or robotic approaches with similar outcomes to the standard approach [21, 22]. Even new approaches such as laparosendoscopic single-site surgery (LESS) are being applied recently in the field of pancreatic surgery [23, 24]. However, there are some limitations that have hindered the wide use of minimally invasive pancreatic surgery, mainly due to the challenges of these kinds of interventions. The retroperitoneal location of the pancreas makes it difficult to reach during surgery. In addition, this glandular organ presents a delicate structure close to major vascular structures. There are also some technical limitations related to minimally invasive surgery (MIS) such as the lack of visual and tactile information. Increasing the capability to visualize tumor margins or to identify small metastatic nodules may significantly improve the surgical procedure to prevent positive resection margins, and therefore, surgical outcomes [25]. Image-guided techniques can provide intraoperative margin assessment and visualization methods, which may be advantageous in guiding the surgeon to achieve curative resections. Some of these emerging modalities are intraoperative near-infrared fluorescence imaging and surgical navigation systems [26, 27]. However, despite the high rate of positive resections in pancreatic surgery, there is limited medical literature regarding the use of navigation systems as a support during pancreatic interventions. In this chapter, the current laparoscopic surgical techniques

and image-guided methods for pancreatic surgery and their associate surgical outcomes will be reviewed.

2. Laparoscopic techniques for pancreatic surgery

Pancreatic cancer is a complex disease, whose optimal treatment depends heavily on careful accurate staging [28]. Surgical resection is still the only potentially curative therapy for pancreatic cancer. However, pancreatic resection is technically challenging and a complex surgical procedure. In this section, the current laparoscopic surgical techniques for pancreatic surgery and their associated surgical outcomes will be reviewed. In order to reach more representative information, only studies published after 2010 and with more than 50 patients included, were taken into account. No limitation in the number of patients was set for the studies using LESS.

2.1. Laparoscopic surgery

2.1.1. Laparoscopic pancreaticoduodenectomy

The first laparoscopic pancreaticoduodenectomy (LPD) was published by Gagner and Pomp in 1994 [29]. They concluded that, although technically feasible, this approach did not confer significant benefit over the conventional open approach in terms of postoperative outcomes or reduced postoperative recovery period. One of the largest barriers of this complex procedure is the reconstruction phase due to the three separate anastomoses to be performed (pancreaticojejunostomy, hepaticojejunostomy, and gastrojejunostomy).

	N	Conv. (%)	Time (min)	EBL (ml)	LHS (days)	Morb. (%)	Mort. (%)	PF (%)	LN (%)	R0 (%)
[30]	53	17	541	195	8	77.3	5.7	13.2	44.2	94.9
[31]	384				10		5.2		4.7	80
[32]	983						5. 1			
[33]	108		379.4	492.4	6					
[34]	65	4.6	368	240	7	40	1.5	16.9	23.1	89
[35]	105	4.7	487.3		15	25	0.9	5.7	12.4	100
[36]	96	3.1					0	28.1		
[37]	75	13.3	551		7	31		9.3		
[38]	137		480.4	592	14.1					
[39]	681				9	39.4	3.8			

N: number of patients; Conv.: conversions; EBL: estimated blood loss; LHS: length of hospital stay; Morb.: morbidity rate; Mort.: mortality rate; PF: pancreatic fistulas; LN: lymph nodes; R0: R0 resection rate.

Table 1. Reported outcomes in laparoscopic pancreaticoduodenectomy.

A summary of the outcomes reported for LPDs are presented in **Table 1**. The average operation time was 486.7 min (range 368–551 min), 8.5% (range 3–17%) conversions, 342.3 ml (range 195–

http://dx.doi.org/10.5772/66171

592 ml) blood loss, 8.9 days (range 6–15 days) hospital stay, 32% (range 25–40%) morbidity, 2.6% (range 0–5%) mortality, 14.7% (range 6–28%) pancreatic fistulas, 21.1% (range 6–28%) harvested lymph nodes, and 89.7% (range 80–100%) R0 resection. The highest rate of conversions reported was due to suspected portal vein involvement [30]. Regarding morbidity rates, the highest rate was caused mainly by surgical site infection, postoperative pancreatic fistula, and intraabdominal access [30]. Myocardial infarctions and positive margins were the main mortality causes [30, 31]. Comparing these results with the conventional open approach [16], LPD leads to an increase in operating time, rate of pancreatic fistulas, and R0 resections; a decrease in estimated blood loss and harvested lymph nodes; and similar results in length of hospital stay, morbidity, and mortality rates.

Most of the studies reported longer operation times using the laparoscopic approach compared to the open approach [30, 35, 37]. Although some studies reported comparable outcomes between open and LPD [30], in general, reduction of blood loss and hospital stay [33, 34] are shown for LPD. In some studies, LPD was associated with equivalent overall hospital cost compared with open pancreaticoduodenectomy [37, 39]. While operating time and supply costs were higher for LPD, it was balanced by reduced cost due to the shorter postoperative hospital stay. A steep learning curve is another aspect associated with LDP and some researchers stated that this procedure should be performed in centers by surgeons with substantial knowledge, experience, and skills [34, 36].

2.1.2. Laparoscopic distal pancreatectomy

Laparoscopic distal pancreatectomy (LDP) was first reported in 1996 by Gagner and Cuschieri [40, 41]. During this intervention, the tail of the pancreas or the tail and a portion of the body of the pancreas are removed. In some cases, the spleen is also removed. This operation is used more often to treat pancreatic NETs found in the tail and body of the pancreas. The determination of resectability is often based on the extent of involvement of the celiac axis [42].

A summary of the outcomes for LDPs are shown in **Table 2**. In brief, the average operation time was 215.2 min, 12% conversion rate, 241.7 ml estimated blood loss, 7.6 days length of hospital stay, 32.5% morbidity rate, 0.3% mortality rate, 21.2% pancreatic fistulas, 10.2% harvested lymph nodes, 89.5% R0 resection, and 46.3% spleen-preserving rate. Comparing these results with the outcomes from conventional open surgery [43, 44], there is a decrease in operation time, estimated blood loss, length of hospital stay, and mortality rate; similar morbidity rates; and an increased rate of pancreatic fistulas and spleen preservation.

Satisfactory oncological outcomes have been reported for LDP in patients with PDA and left-side pancreatic neoplasms [58, 61]. Although some studies reported similar outcomes as open distal pancreatectomy [21], most of the studies reported a clear reduction of blood loss [50, 53, 62, 63, 65] and hospital stay [45, 48, 50, 53, 31, 59, 61–65]. An increase in quality of life is reported when compared to the conventional approach [46]. Similar costs for the laparoscopic and open approaches are reported [63]. The increased OR cost associated with LDP is often offset by the shorter hospitalization and lower overall cost of postoperative care [57].

Regarding the spleen-preserving rate, results stated that it is worth to attempt laparoscopic spleen-preserving DP in patients with a presumed benign to borderline tumor of the body-tail of the pancreas [54]. The most positive results were reported for the splenic vessels preservation technique regarding the conservation of the spleen [51, 66].

	N	Conv. (%)	Time (min)	EBL (ml)	LHS (days)	Morb. (%)	Mort. (%)	PF (%)	LN (%)	R0 (%)	SP (%)
[21]	64	32.8	213	275	8	16		11	8	62	79.6
[45]	535	22.8			7		0		15	86	
[46]	100	23	239	464	7.7	66	0	53		73.3	
[47]	94							0	11		
[48]	71	9.1	250	150	5	28.2	0	11		97.2	15.5
[49]	67	14.9	203	100	6	21	1.5	19	6		
[50]	107	30	193	150	5	27	0	15		97	21
[51]* †	55	9	214.7	342.8	8.2	27.3	0	16			93.4
[51]* †	85	13	199.2	288.9	10.5	38.8	0	26	3		84.7
[52]	132	6.1	156.5	197.4	6	43.2	0.8	21	8	96.2	9.8
[53]	131	31.3	193	262	5	32	0	8	11	100	22.1
[54]	100	2	207		8.7	49	0	27		98	41
[55]	143	5.6	236	334				17			
[56]	902	6.4	316	243	18.9	23.6		66	11		32
[57]	70	7.1	145	113	5.8	49	0	36	5		
[58]	196	2.5	220	250	8	31.9	0	24	10	83.8	
[59]	144	39.5			6.8		0		17	87	
[60]	70	7.1	239		9	25.7	0	19	3	75.7	
[61]	359		195		8	12	0	28	20	91.6	49.6
[62]	82	7	188	70	4	32.9	0	13		97	12
[63]	100	4	214	171	6.1	34	3	17	15	100	25
[64]	73	15	352		5	40	0	22		97	
[65]	45	0	158.7	122.6	7.9	26.7		16			53.3
[66]†	70	0	220	352	10.4	32.9	0	17			100
[67]* †	246	0	193.4	378	8.2	32.5	0	20			54.8
[67]* †	203	0	204.4	328	7.7	25	0	4			

N: number of patients; Conv.: conversions; EBL: estimated blood loss; LHS: length of hospital stay; Morb.: morbidity rate; Mort.: mortality rate; PF: pancreatic fistulas; LN: lymph nodes; R0: R0 resection rate; SP: spleen preserving.
*Two groups.
†Spleen-preserving DP.

Table 2. Reported outcomes in laparoscopic distal pancreatectomy.

With growing surgical experience and refinement in the surgical technique, the indications for LDP have substantially broadened [52]. In this sense, the learning curve appeared to have been completed after 17 procedures [68], but strict selection criteria, high-volume hospital, and experienced team in open pancreatic surgery may play an important role in shortening this learning curve [69].

2.2. Laparoendoscopic single-site surgery

Recent interest in improving cosmetic outcomes has led to laparoendoscopic single-site surgery (LESS) being performed in a variety of procedures. In this sense, LESS is now consolidated as a real alternative to conventional laparoscopic surgery, with numerous studies sustaining its feasibility and therapeutic safety. However, single-site pancreatectomy has been explored and described only in recent years, and therefore, literature is limited to DP procedures and mostly to single case reports or small case series, as it is considered to be a challenging procedure. Only one study has been found for a PD through the single-site approach [70]. In this case, a surgical resection for a malignant melanoma metastatic to the pancreas was performed. The resection was carried out preserving the pylorus. No detailed information about the intervention and surgical outcomes were reported.

	N	Conv. (%)	Time (min)	EBL (ml)	LHS (days)	Morb. (%)	Mort. (%)	PF (%)	LN (%)	R0 (%)	SP (%)
[23]	20		176		2	4	20	20	0	100	90
[24]	14	7.1	166.4	157.1	7.6	0	7.1	0			50
[71]	1	0	330	100	7	1		100	0	100	0
[72]	1	0	170		5		0			100	0
[73]†	1	0	233	<100	3		0			100	100
[74]	12	20	279.8	185	12.2	3	41.6	25		100	33.3
[75]	8	0	145	225	6	2	50	25		100	62.5
[76]*	2	0	232.5	100	7, 5		0	100			
[77]	1	0			5	0			0	100	0

N: number of patients; Conv.: conversions; EBL: estimated blood loss; LHS: length of hospital stay; Morb.: morbidity rate; Mort.: mortality rate; PF: pancreatic fistulas; LN: lymph nodes; R0: R0 resection rate; SP: spleen preserving.
*Two groups.
†Spleen-preserving DP.

Table 3. Reported outcomes in single-site distal pancreatectomy.

The average operation time reported for LESS distal pancreatectomy (**Table 3**) was 218 min (range 145–330 min), 3% (range 0–20%) conversion rate, 144 ml (range 100–225 ml) estimated blood loss, 6 days (range 2–12 days) length of hospital stay, 15% (range 0–50%) morbidity, 0% mortality, 100% R0 resection, and 42% (range 0–100) spleen-preserving rate. Comparing the results with the conventional laparoscopic approach, there is a decreased rate of conversions, estimated blood loss, length of hospital stay, and morbidity; a similar mortality rate; increased average of pancreatic fistulas and R0 resections; and lower spleen-preserving rate.

Barbaros et al. [71] reported the first transumbilical laparoscopic single-site DP in a patient with metastatic lesions on the pancreas. The patient developed a pancreatic fistula. Haugvik et al. [75] compared the results of 8 single-incision DPs with 16 conventional LDPs. They reported no significant differences in operative time, intraoperative bleeding, resection status, and hospital stay between the two groups. Four surgical complications were reported for LESS

and five for the conventional approach, including two patients for each group who developed a pancreatic fistula. There was no conversion to conventional laparoscopic or open surgery in any procedure. No differences between operative and postoperative results were also obtained by Yao et al. [24], who compared the surgical outcomes of 14 transumbilical laparoscopic single-site DPs with seven conventional multiport interventions. One conversion to open surgery and one case of leakage were reported for the LESS interventions. Machado et al. [23] reported 4 cases of pancreatic fistula in a study of 20 DPs. Some cases reported no surgical complications during the intervention [72, 76]. In a case study without using any commercial surgical port for LESS [77], the patient developed fever and leukocytosis after surgery. Bracale et al. [72] presented the first LESS DP for an adenocarcinoma. They reported no postoperative complications after 4 months follow-up.

Spleen preservation is an important issue in patients undergoing DP. However, only a few studies have reported spleen preservation through LESS. Chang et al. [73] reported a case of ransumbilical LESS spleen-preserving DP for a cystic tumor in the body of the pancreas. No surgical complications were reported. In another study, Han et al. [74] compared the results from 12 LESS DPs to 28 cases using a conventional laparoscopic approach. The mean surgery time and hospital stay in the LESS group were significantly longer. The spleen preservation was possible in 60.7% of the patients who underwent the conventional approach and 33.3% for the LESS. No significant differences in intraoperative blood loss, tumor size, conversion rate, and postoperative complications between the two groups were found.

In general, authors stated that single-site laparoscopic PD is a feasible and safe technique [23, 72, 74], which can be successfully performed in selected cases and qualified centers [71, 73]. However, they also stated that it is a very demanding procedure with a steep learning curve [74].

2.3. Robotic surgery

Robotic platforms, as the da Vinci® Surgical System (Intuitive Surgical, Sunnyvale, CA, USA), try to overcome many of the key shortcomings of traditional laparoscopy that include monocular vision, limited degrees of freedom, and the effects of pivot and fulcrum, which make complex tasks difficult to master. However, there are also some drawbacks regarding the use of these systems such as the lack of tactile feedback and their cost, including maintenance. Since its first reported application in 2003 [78], the application of robotic technology in pancreatic interventions has been increasing. The main benefit of robotic-assisted PD in comparison with LPD may be the ease of intracorporeal reconstruction after a long resection [78].

In the scientific literature, most of the studies regarding the robotic-assisted PD and DP are retrospective reviews and case reports (**Table 4** and **5**). The average operation time reported for robot-assisted PD (**Table 4**) was 489.1 min (range 410–568 min), 10% (range 0–22%) conversion rate, 324 ml (range 250–400 ml) estimated blood loss, 13.4 days (range 9–22 days) hospital stay, 48.6% (range 21–67%) morbidity rate, 3.8% (range 1–7%) mortality rate, 17.4% (range 7–30) pancreatic fistulas, 29% (range 11–70%) harvested lymph nodes, and 91% (range 87–95%) R0 resection. Comparing the results with conventional laparoscopic approach,

http://dx.doi.org/10.5772/66171

operative time, length of hospital stay, and negative resections margins are similar; the rate of conversions, morbidity, mortality, and pancreatic fistulas are increased. Positive results have been obtained for robotic-assisted PD in patients with aberrant or anomalous hepatic arterial anatomy [22]. In a prospective analysis with 150 patients, Polanco et al. [79] concluded that larger body mass index, higher EBL, smaller tumor size and smaller duct diameter are the main predictors of postoperative PF in robot-assisted PD. It appears that the learning curve for robot-assisted PD is attained within 80 cases [80].

	N	Conv. (%)	Time (min)	EBL (ml)	LHS (days)	Morb. (%)	Mort. (%)	PF (%)	LN (%)	R0 (%)
[22]*	112	0	500	250	9.5	63.3	6.7	7	20	92.6
[79]	150	7.3	515	300				17		
[80]	200	6.5	483	250	9	67.5	3.3	17	11	92
[84]	60		410	400	20	35	1.7	13	23	94.7
[85]	50	22	421	394	22			30	70	90
[86]	50	16	568	350	10	56	2	20	36	89
[87]	132	8.3	527	>400	10	21	5.3	17	14	87.7

N: number of patients; Conv.: conversions; EBL: estimated blood loss; LHS: length of hospital stay; Morb.: morbidity rate; Mort.: mortality rate; PF: pancreatic fistulas; LN: lymph nodes; R0: R0 resection rate; SP: spleen preserving.
*Two groups.

Table 4. Reported outcomes in robotic-assisted pancreaticoduodenectomy.

	N	Conv. (%)	Time (min)	EBL (ml)	LHS (days)	Morb. (%)	Mort. (%)	PF (%)	LN (%)	R0 (%)	SP (%)
[45]	535	23			7				3	86	
[82]	100	2	246	150		72	0	42	13	95.7	
[83]	55	0	278.2		12.6	61.8	0	53	58	100	61.8
[87]	83	2.4	256	>200	6	13	0	43	17	97	
[88]†	69	0	150	100	11.6	40.6	0	25	22	100	65.2

N: number of patients; Conv.: conversions; EBL: estimated blood loss; LHS: length of hospital stay; Morb.: morbidity rate; Mort.: mortality rate; PF: pancreatic fistulas; LN: lymph nodes; R0: R0 resection rate; SP: spleen preserving.
†Spleen-preserving DP.

Table 5. Reported outcomes in robotic-assisted distal pancreatectomy.

Regarding robot-assisted DP, the average operation time was 232.6 min (range 150–278 min), 5.5% (range 0–23%) conversion rate, 125 ml (range 100–150 ml) estimated blood loss, 9.3 days (range 6–13 days) hospital stay, 46.9% (range 13–72%) morbidity rate, 0% mortality rate, 40.7% (range 24–53%) pancreatic fistula, 22.6% (range 3–58%) harvested lymph nodes, 95.7% (range 86–100%) R0 resection, and 63.5% (range 62–65%) spleen-preserving rate. Comparing these

results with the conventional laparoscopic approach, there is a decreased conversion rate and EBL; and increased operation time, length of hospital stay, morbidity, rate of pancreatic fistulas, R0 resections, and spleen-preserving rate. Morbid obesity and technical difficulty seem to be the two most common reasons for conversion from robotic-assisted hepatobiliary and pancreatic surgery [81]. It appears that the learning curve for robot-assisted DP is approximately 10–40 cases [82, 83].

3. Image-guided techniques for pancreatic surgery

In order to cope with some of the limitations in MIS and guide the surgeon during the surgical procedure, image-guided techniques have been developed. The lack of tactile feedback and 3D sensation in video-assisted surgery accelerated the need for these techniques. In addition, for the human eye, several pathologies, such as the presence of nonsuperficial tumors, are not easily distinguishable from surrounding normal tissue. This makes, in some occasions, decision-making during surgery a very difficult process. During image-guided surgery, diagnostic imaging is used in conjunction with images from the operative field to improve the localization and targeting of pathologies, as well as to monitor and control treatments. The combination of tracking technologies for recording the position of the patient and the surgical instruments with preoperative and intraoperative images provides a comprehensive assistance tool for guiding any MIS intervention [27, 89–91]. Image-guided technology allows for more precise and accurate procedures, allowing surgeons to decide the best approach to address a specific disease before the intervention [92].

Radical surgical resection of tumor tissue is currently the best chance for cure. However, this option is only suitable for a minority of patients, and surgical procedures are complex with high rates of local recurrence. The presence of microscopic residual tumor tissue at the resection margins is one of the main prognostic factors, and therefore optimizing the surgical procedure to prevent positive resection margins is of the utmost importance. Accordingly, intraoperative margin assessment and visualization techniques, as well as image-guided techniques may be advantageous in guiding the surgeon to achieve curative resections.

3.1. Laparoscopic ultrasound (LUS)

Advances in technology over the last 30 years have seen the application of laparoscopic ultrasound (LUS) expand beyond its initial limited diagnostic role to assisting in tumor staging, guiding intervention, locating lesions intraoperatively, assessing anatomic relationships, and in directed therapy [93–95]. The main application of LUS during pancreatic and liver surgery is providing real-time imaging guidance for resectability assessment and detection of vessel involvement, aiming to decrease the number of irradical resections [95]. The reported overall sensitivity, specificity, and accuracy of combined diagnostic laparoscopy and LUS in predicting resectability has been reported to be 100, 91, and 96%, respectively [96]. LUS should be considered for confirmation of staging of disease when there is a strong suspicion of unresectability and tumor borders are not clearly defined by CT scan [96].

http://dx.doi.org/10.5772/66171

LUS plays an integral part in the management of cystic lesions of the pancreas, particularly the characterization of suspected intraductal papillary mucinous neoplasms (IPMNs) [95, 97, 98]. IPMNs appear as well-defined hypoechoic masses with associated posterior enhancement. The malignant potential of IPMNs is directly related to its relationship with the main pancreatic duct and adjacent blood vessels (**Figure 1**). LUS allows defining the cysts borders (**Figure 2**) and evaluating the relationship of the lesion with the main duct and any major vessels [95, 98, 99].

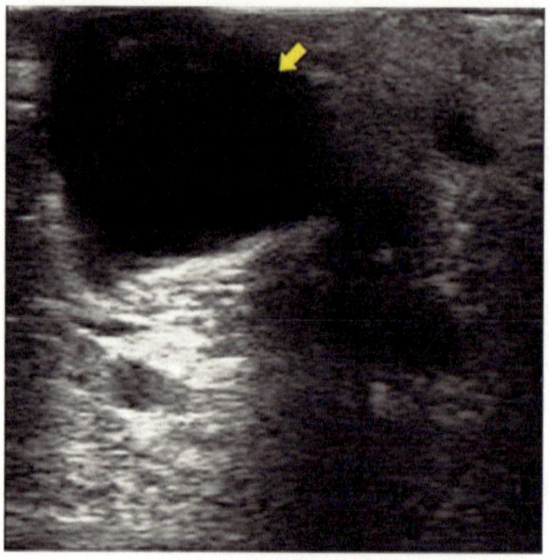

Figure 2. LUS image of a pancreatic cystic tumor. The lesion appears as a hypoechoic mass (yellow arrow).

In the case of pancreatic adenocarcinomas, they appear as a homogeneous hypoechoic mass with poorly defined margins. Large tumors can display a mixed echogenicity. A sensitivity of 90% for assessing positive lymph nodes and 100% for venous invasion have been reported for laparoscopy combined with LUS examination [100]. Regarding NETs, LUS facilitates intraoperative decision-making and demonstrates anatomic details, such as the tumor location and its relation to the adjacent vascular structures and main pancreatic duct [95, 97]. In ultrasound images, NETs typically appear as well-defined, homogeneous, and hypoechoic masses [93]. Findings from LUS inspection help to decide whether to perform either tumor enucleation or resection during laparoscopic intervention [93].

3.2. Fluorescence

Near-infrared (NIR) light (700–900 nm) is a novel imaging technique that can penetrate through several millimeters even centimeters of tissue, revealing targets below the tissue surface [101]. This imaging modality does not use ionizing radiation or direct tissue contact, making it a remarkably safe technique. NIR fluorescent contrast agents can be visualized with acquisition times in the millisecond range, enabling real-time guidance during surgery. Furthermore, as NIR light is invisible to the human eye, it does not alter the look of the surgical field, thus minimizing the learning curve [102]. The main aim of this imaging modality is to fill the gap between preoperative imaging and intraoperative reality.

Fluorescence-guided systems provide an additional tool for diagnosis of pancreatic cancer, real-time image guidance during tumor resection, and inspection to confirm complete resection [103]. This intraoperative modality can assist surgeons to visualize tumors, sentinel lymph nodes, and vital structures in real time [102]. This technology could represent the next step to improving treatment of pancreatic cancer in laparoscopic resections. However, most of the published studies for pancreatic surgery are limited to animal models.

Two main components are needed for fluorescence-guided surgery, fluorescent contrast agents and a NIR camera system. Several intraoperative NIR fluorescence camera systems have been developed for both open and laparoscopic surgery, some of which are commercially available and Food and Drug Administration (FDA) approved [104]. Fluorescent contrast agents contain a fluorescent component (fluorophore), which emits NIR fluorescent light after being excited with a NIR light source. Visualization of the tissue is based on the signal of the contrast agent in the region of interest relative to the background signal, known as signal-to-background ratio.

Indocyanine green (ICG) and methylene blue (MB) are the only NIR fluorophores that are registered with the FDA and the European Medicines Agency for clinical use. ICG emits fluorescent light at ≈800 nm and it is cleared rapidly by the liver and almost exclusively excreted into the bile, permitting imaging of bile ducts. MB has been applied clinically for many years as a visible contrast agent, and when diluted to levels that are almost undetectable to the human eye, MB becomes a fluorophore emitting at ≈700 nm. MB is cleared equally by both liver and kidney, permitting imaging of both bile ducts and ureters. ICG has been shown to accumulate around hepatic metastasis of pancreatic and colorectal cancers [105]. Methylene blue tends to accumulate in NETs after high-dose intra-arterial injection [103, 106]. The chemical structures of both ICG and MB do not allow these agents to be conjugated to tissue-specific, therefore, they are nonspecific NIR contrast agents [102, 107].

Applications of this technique during hepatopancreatobiliary surgery include tumor imaging in liver and pancreas, and real-time imaging of the biliary tree. Pessaux et al. [26] presented a robotic pancreaticoduodenectomy assisted by fluorescence imaging, providing enhanced visualization of the common bile and cystic ducts during the intervention (**Figure 1**). Subar et al. [108] reported a case of a LPD to treat an ampullary lesion in the duodenum. Before the pancreaticojejunostomy, the viability of the margin of the remnant pancreas was assessed with NIR imaging. The NIR technique improved the detection of ischemic tissue of the pancreatic margin after resection. This may lead to an increase in blood supply to the pancreatic anastomosis, and therefore potentially help to decrease the incidence of pancreatic fistulas.

In a study with different pancreatic tumors on three experimental porcine models, we analyzed the usefulness of NIR imaging during laparoscopic pancreaticoduodenectomy and single-site distal pancreatectomy procedures. In two animals, a tumor model was created in the head of the pancreas. In the third animal, the tumor model was developed in the tail of the pancreas. NIR imaging was used as guidance during LPD and LESS distal pancreatectomy. The patency of the hepaticojejunostomy was assessed by means of ICG excretion and fluoroscopic imaging. During surgery, identification of the biliary anatomy and vascular anatomy of the pancreas was possible in all procedures using NIR imaging (**Figure 3**). Biliary excretion of ICG was not clearly visualized during the patency test, but fluoroscopic imaging was positive in one case.

http://dx.doi.org/10.5772/66171

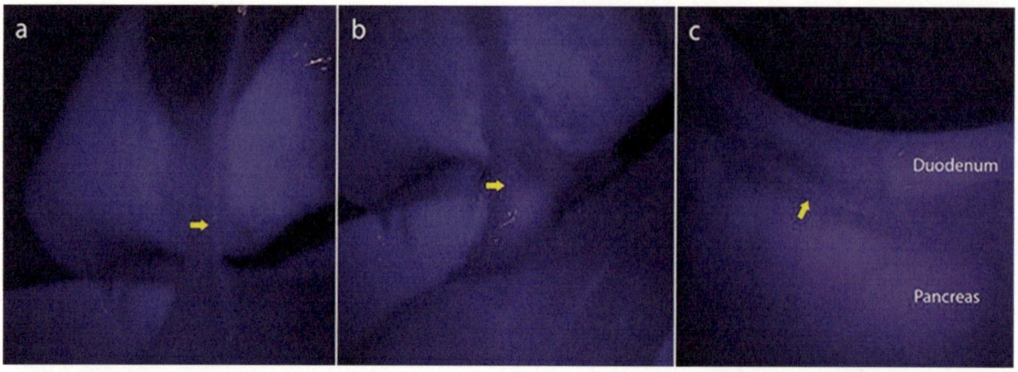

Figure 3. NIR image of biliary and pancreatic anatomy: Cystic artery (a, yellow arrow), cystic duct (b, yellow arrow), and pancreaticoduodenal artery (c, yellow arrow).

To obtain the full advantage of NIR fluorescence imaging for pancreatic cancer visualization, such as tumor imaging, tumor specific NIR conjugated agents need to be designed and tested. The tumor-targeting capability of the fluorophore-conjugated anticarcinoembryonic antigen antibody has been demonstrated in orthotopic models for intraoperative tumor visualization of both primary and metastatic deposits of pancreatic cancer [25, 109]. Metildi et al. [109] concluded that mice treated with fluorescence-guided laparoscopic surgery permitted adequate labeling and distinction of tumor margins before tumor resection, decreasing local recurrence, and increasing survival compared to mice treated with standard bright-light laparoscopic surgery.

3.3. Surgical navigation

Surgical navigation systems (SNS) combine preoperative and intraoperative image information with position and orientation tracking of surgical instruments during the surgical intervention as a surgical decision-making tool helping to improve the safety, accuracy, and efficiency of surgeries [27, 91, 92]. In MIS, due to surgeon having less visual and tactile perception compared to open surgery, image assistance becomes extensively helpful for 3D understanding of the surgical scenario and localization of lesion and essential anatomic structures.

The basic setup of a SNS consists of a preoperative image data (typically MR and CT), a tracking system (mainly electromagnetic or optical), a computer platform with screen, and the respective navigation software [89]. The combination of image-guided surgery with navigation technology consists of several steps, which are critical to ensure safety and accuracy of a procedure [27]: (1) acquisition of preoperative images and visualization for optimal diagnosis and planning, (2) accurate registration of preoperative data to the patient coordinate space and visualization in the OR, (3) intraoperative image acquisition and visualization/fusion with the preoperative images to update for anatomical shifts, and (4) postoperative imaging and visualization for evaluation of the surgical treatment.

Despite the use of navigation systems, abdominal surgery is still a challenging task. Commercial SNS are available for resection and ablation procedures of the liver (example: CAScination AG, Switzerland). However, to the best of our knowledge, no commercial systems are available or studies in the scientific literature have been published regarding the use of SNS for assistance during pancreatic cancer surgery.

We were recently able to demonstrate the usefulness of the CustusX navigation system for image guidance during a patient case, a distal pancreatectomy for the resection of a cystic tumor in the body of the pancreas (unpublished case). CustusX is an open-source navigation research platform for image-guided interventions [91]. This platform has been successfully used for many clinical applications such as neurosurgery, spine procedures, bronchoscopy, endovascular therapy, and laparoscopic procedures like adrenalectomy and lately for liver and pancreas surgery [91, 110–112].

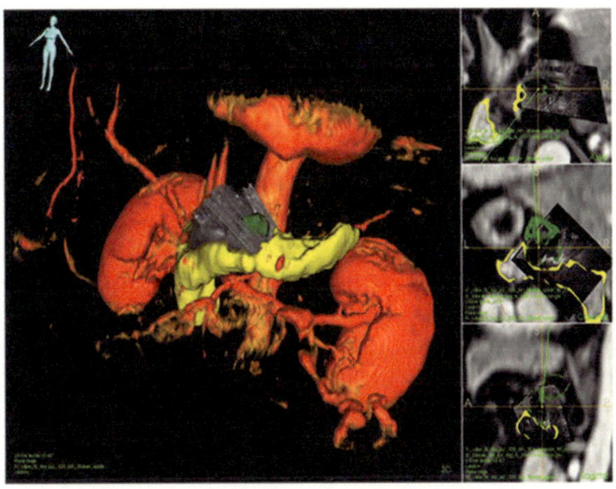

Figure 4. Snapshot of the CustusX platform during a distal pancreatectomy. The tumor is shown in green and the pancreas in yellow. The US imaging is superimposed on the 3D model from a preoperative MRI scan.

Prior to surgery, MR and CT images were acquired and imported into the navigation system software for reconstruction into 3D. The anatomical structures of interest, including the pancreas, tumor, and vessels were segmented semiautomatically [112]. The navigation system was integrated with a LUS probe running on an ultrasound scanner (Ultrasonix, Canada) with digital research interface to the navigation system. The probe was tracked by an electromagnetic sensor integrated in the tip. A probe calibration was carried out in a laboratory using a robotic arm and a well-defined geometric structure in a water tank [113]. An intraoperative registration procedure was carried out to combine the intraoperative LUS with the corresponding preoperative MR and CT images, displaying them simultaneously (**Figure 4**). This enabled the location of the lesion based on multimodal display, providing a useful tool for the surgeons to identify the anatomical structures of interest, meet their relation to other adjacent structures, and define safely and accurately the resection margin during the course of the distal pancreatectomy.

3.4. Augmented reality

Another available technology for intraoperative surgical guidance is augmented reality (AR). In surgery, AR is the fusion of artificial computer-generated images (3D virtual model) generally obtained from preoperative medical imaging and real-time patient images with the aim to visualize unapparent anatomical details. This results in the visualization of internal structures through overlying tissues, providing a virtual transparent vision of surgical anatomy. Potential advantages of the use of this imaging technology in surgery include the delineation of dissection planes or resection margins and the avoidance of injury to invisible structures.

The registration process is one of the main challenges of AR, in which the virtual model and intraoperative images should be merged in real time. In this sense, intraoperative accuracy is highly affected by mobile or deformable structures due to the heartbeat, ventilation, or laparoscopic insufflation.

A method to overlay anatomical information from preoperative CT studies onto the patient's body surface during gastrointestinal, hepatobiliary, and pancreatic surgery was presented by Sugimoto et al. [114]. For enabling the simultaneous display of the gastrointestinal tract and pancreatobiliary duct with associated blood vessels, a carbon dioxide-enhanced virtual multiple detector CT cholangiopancreatography was performed. Manual registration based on physiological markers was used. However, this method does not deal with possible alteration of the patient anatomy during the course of the surgery. A robotic pancreaticoduodenectomy assisted by AR was presented by Pessaux et al. [26]. In this study, a 3D virtual model of the patient from a preoperative CT scan was manually merged with the stereoscopic images from the da Vinci® robotic system.

4. Conclusions

Pancreatic cancer has a high mortality rate and, at the time of diagnosis, the number of patients with potentially resectable tumors is considerably low. Surgery is still the only viable option for treatment of pancreatic cancer. However, surgical procedures for pancreatic resection are complex and require high surgical expertise. Pancreatic tumors can be treated through laparoscopic surgery with similar outcomes to the conventional approach. In general, studies reported that minimally invasive pancreatic surgery is feasible, safe, and with a steep learning curve. Laparoscopic procedures reported a reduction of blood loss, length of hospital stay, and positive resection margins, as well as an improvement in spleen-preserving rates when compared to open surgery. Laparoendoscopic single-site surgery reduces the blood loss and morbidity, compared with the conventional laparoscopic approach. In robot-assisted pancreatic surgery, reported surgical outcomes are similar to laparoscopic surgery, with an apparent increase in the splenic preservation rate and negative resection margins.

Laparoscopic pancreatic surgery has some technical limitations for the surgeon such as the reduced tactile and visual information. Besides, intraoperative tumor identification may be a

challenging task in some cases due to the anatomical location of the pancreas, nearby major vascular structures, and frequently inflamed surrounding pancreatic tissue. These limitations may significantly impact the surgical procedure to prevent positive resection margins. Image-guided techniques provide intraoperative margin assessment and visualization methods, which may be advantageous in guiding the surgeon to achieve curative resections, resulting in improved surgical outcomes. Reported cases of fluorescence-guided pancreatic surgery showed that this imaging technique could be beneficial in surgeries where the pancreatic anatomy is difficult to identify. Navigation systems combine preoperative and intraoperative imaging, providing location of the anatomical structures of interest with respect to surgical instruments as well as the extent of the tumor to be addressed, which allows for a safe and precise definition of resection margins. Thus, surgeons will have a comprehensive system to support and guide pancreatic surgeries, with the ultimate goal of improving surgical outcomes and increase the rate of negative resections and the subsequent positive effect on the life expectancy of the patient.

Acknowledgements

This study was supported by the Norwegian National Advisory Unit for Ultrasound and Image-Guided Therapy (St. Olav's Hospital, NTNU, SINTEF); SINTEF; St. Olavs University Hospital; Liaison Committee between the Central Norway Regional Health Authority (RHA); the Norwegian University of Science and Technology (NTNU); the Extremadura Region Government, Spain; and the European Social Fund (PO14034).

Author details

Juan A. Sánchez-Margallo[1,2], Thomas Langø[2,3*], Erlend F. Hofstad[2,3], Ronald Mårvik[3,4] and Francisco M. Sánchez-Margallo[5]

*Address all correspondence to: thomasl@sintef.no

1 Department of Medical Technology, SINTEF, Trondheim, Norway

2 Department of Computer Systems and Telematics Engineering, University of Extremadura, Badajoz, Spain

3 Norwegian National Advisory Unit on Ultrasound and Image-Guided Therapy, St. Olavs Hospital, Trondheim University Hospital, Trondheim, Norway

4 Department of Gastrointestinal Surgery, St. Olavs Hospital, Trondheim University Hospital, Trondheim, Norway

5 Jesús Usón Minimally Invasive Surgery Centre, Cáceres, Spain

References

[1] Fitzmaurice C, Dicker D, Pain A, Hamavid H, Moradi-Lakeh M, MacIntyre MF, et al. The global burden of cancer 2013. JAMA Oncol. 2015; 1(4): 505–27.

[2] Malvezzi M, Bertuccio P, Levi F, La Vecchia C, Negri E. European cancer mortality predictions for the year 2013. Ann Oncol. 2013; 24: 792–800.

[3] Siegel RL, Miller KD, Jemal A. Cancer statistics, 2015. CA Cancer J Clin. 2015; 65(1): 5–29.

[4] Howlader N, Noone AM, Krapcho M, Garshell J, Miller D, Altekruse SF, et al. SEER Cancer Statistics Review, 1975–2013. Bethesda, MD: National Cancer Institute. 2016.

[5] Ryan DP, Hong TS, Bardeesy N. Pancreatic adenocarcinoma. N Engl J Med. 2014; 371(11): 1039–49.

[6] ACS, American Cancer Society. Pancreatic Cancer. 2015. Available at: http://www.cancer.org/cancer/pancreaticcancer/detailedguide/pancreatic-cancer-pdf

[7] Eurostat. Causes of death—Deaths by country of residence and occurrence [Internet]. 2015. Available at: http://appsso.eurostat.ec.europa.eu/nui/submitViewTableAction.do

[8] Ferlay J, Steliarova-Foucher E, Lortet-Tieulent J, Rosso S, Coebergh JWW, Comber H, et al. Cancer incidence and mortality patterns in Europe: Estimates for 40 countries in 2012. Eur J Cancer. 2013; 49(6):1374–403.

[9] Harris RE. Epidemiology of pancreatic cancer. In: Harris RE, editor. Epidemiology of Chronic Disease. Burlington: Jones & Bartlett. 2013. pp. 181–90.

[10] Hamilton SR, Aaltonen LA. Tumours of the exocrine pancreas. In: Hamilton SR, Aaltonen LA, editors. World Health Organization Classification of Tumours: Pathology and Genetics of Tumours of the Digestive System. Lyon: IARC Press. 2000. pp. 219–50.

[11] Jacobs EJ, Chanock SJ, Fuchs CS, Lacroix A, McWilliams RR, Steplowski E, et al. Family history of cancer and risk of pancreatic cancer: a pooled analysis from the Pancreatic Cancer Cohort Consortium (PanScan). Int J Cancer. 2010; 127(6): 1421–8.

[12] Chen YJ, Wu SC, Chen CY, Tzou SC, Cheng TL, Huang YF, et al. Peptide-based MRI contrast agent and near-infrared fluorescent probe for intratumoral legumain detection. Biomaterials. 2014; 35: 304–15.

[13] Vincent A, Herman J, Schulick R, Hruban RH, Goggins M. Pancreatic cancer. Lancet. 2011; 378: 607–20.

[14] Hidalgo M. Pancreatic cancer. N Engl J Med. 2010; 362: 1605–17.

[15] Konstantinidis IT, Warshaw AL, Allen JN, Blaszkowsky LS, Castillo CF, Deshpande V, et al. Pancreatic ductal adenocarcinoma: is there a survival difference for R1 resections

versus locally advanced unresectable tumors? What is a "true" R0 resection? Ann Surg. 2013; 257(4):731–6.

[16] Winter JM, Cameron JL, Campbell KA, Arnold MA, Chang DC, Coleman J, et al. 1423 pancreaticoduodenectomies for pancreatic cancer: A single-institution experience. J Gastrointest Surg. 2006; 10:1199–210.

[17] Willett CG, Lewandrowski K, Warshaw AL, Efird J, Compton CC. Resection margins in carcinoma of the head of the pancreas. Implications for radiation therapy. Ann Surg. 1993; 217: 144–8.

[18] Garcea G, Dennison AR, Pattenden CJ, Neal CP, Sutton CD, Berry DP. Survival following curative resection for pancreatic ductal adenocarcinoma. A systematic review of the literature. JOP. 2008; 9: 99–132.

[19] Kato K, Yamada S, Sugimoto H, Kanazumi N, Nomoto S, Takeda S, et al. Prognostic factors for survival after extended pancreatectomy for pancreatic head cancer: influence of resection margin status on survival. Pancreas. 2009; 38(6):605–12.

[20] Andrén-Sandberg A. Prognostic factors in pancreatic cancer. N Am J Med Sci. 2012; 4(1):9–12.

[21] de Rooij T, Jilesen AP, Boerma D, Bonsing BA, Bosscha K, van Dam RM, et al. A nationwide comparison of laparoscopic and open distal pancreatectomy for benign and malignant disease. J Am Coll Surg. 2015; 220(3):263–70.e1

[22] Nguyen TK, Zenati MS, Boone BA, Steve J, Hogg ME, Bartlett DL, et al. Robotic pancreaticoduodenectomy in the presence of aberrant or anomalous hepatic arterial anatomy: safety and oncologic outcomes. HPB. 2015; 17(7):594–9.

[23] Machado MA, Surjan RC, Makdissi FF. Laparoscopic distal pancreatectomy using single-port platform: technique, safety, and feasibility in a clinical case series. J Laparoendosc Adv Surg Tech. 2015; 25(7):581–5.

[24] Yao D, Wu S, Li Y, Chen Y, Yu X, Han J. Transumbilical single-incision laparoscopic distal pancreatectomy: preliminary experience and comparison to conventional multiport laparoscopic surgery. BMC Surg. 2014; 14(1):105.

[25] Cao HST, Kaushal S, Metildi CA, Menen RS, Lee C, Snyder CS, et al. Tumor-specific fluorescence antibody imaging enables accurate staging laparoscopy in an orthotopic model of pancreatic cancer. Hepatogastroenterology. 2011; 29(6):997–1003.

[26] Pessaux P, Diana M, Soler L, Piardi T, Mutter D, Marescaux J. Robotic duodenopancreatectomy assisted with augmented reality and real-time fluorescence guidance. Surg Endosc. 2014; 28(8): 2493–8.

[27] Langø T, Hernes TN, Mårvik R. Navigated ultrasound in laparoscopic surgery. In: Malik A, editor. Advances in Laparoscopic Surgery. Rijeka: InTech. 2012. pp. 77–98.

[28] Harrison EM, Garden OJ. Laparoscopic Ultrasound in Staging of GI Malignancies. Abdominal Ultrasound for Surgeons. New York, NY: Springer New York. 2014. pp. 129–50.

[29] Gagner M, Pomp A. Laparoscopic pylorus-preserving pancreatoduodenectomy. Surg Endosc. 1994; 8: 408e10

[30] Asbun HJ, Stauffer JA. Laparoscopic approach to distal and subtotal pancreatectomy: A clockwise technique. Surg Endosc. 2012; 25(8):2643–9.

[31] Sharpe SM, Talamonti MS, Wang CE, Prinz RA, Roggin KK, Bentrem DJ, et al. Early national experience with laparoscopic pancreaticoduodenectomy for ductal adenocarcinoma:a comparison of laparoscopic pancreaticoduodenectomy and open pancreaticoduodenectomy from the national cancer data base. J Am Coll Surg. 2015; 221(1):175–84.

[32] Abdelgadir AM, Choudhury K, Dinan MA, Reed SD, Scheri RP, Blazer DG, et al. Minimally invasive versus open pancreaticoduodenectomy for cancer: practice patterns and short-term outcomes among 7061 patients. Ann Surg. 2015; 262(2):372–7.

[33] Croome KP, Farnell MB, Que FG, Reid-Lombardo KM, Truty MJ, Nagorney DM. Total laparoscopic pancreaticoduodenectomy for pancreatic ductal adenocarcinoma: Oncologic advantages over open approaches? Ann Surg. 2014; 260(4):633–8.

[34] Kendrick ML, Cusati D.Total laparoscopic pancreaticoduodenectomy. Arch Surg. 2010; 145(1):188–93.

[35] Kim SC, Song KB, Jung YS, Kim YH, Park DH, Lee SSK, et al. Short-term clinical outcomes for 100 consecutive cases of laparoscopic pylorus-preserving pancreatoduodenectomy: improvement with surgical experience. Surg Endosc. 2013; 27(1):95–103.

[36] Machado MAC, Surjan RCT, Goldman SM, Ardengh JC, Makdissi FF. Laparoscopic pancreatic resection. From enucleation to pancreatoduodenectomy. 11-year experience. Arq Gastroenterol. 2013; 50(3):214–8.

[37] Mesleh MG, Stauffer JA, Bowers SP, Asbun HJ. Cost analysis of open and laparoscopic pancreaticoduodenectomy: A single institution comparison. Surg Endosc. 2013;27(12): 4518–23.

[38] Song KB, Kim SC, Hwang DW, Lee JH, Lee DJ, Lee JW, et al. Matched case-control analysis comparing laparoscopic and open pylorus-preserving pancreaticoduodenectomy in patients with periampullary tumors. Ann Surg. 2015; 262(1):146–55.

[39] Tran TB, Dua MM, Worhunsky DJ, Poultsides GA, Norton JA, Visser BC. The first decade of laparoscopic pancreaticoduodenectomy in the United States: costs and outcomes using the nationwide inpatient sample. Surg Endosc. 2016; 30(5):1778–83.

[40] Gagner M, Pomp A, Herrera MF. Early experience with laparoscopic resections of islet cell tumors. Surgery. 1996; 120: 1051–4.

[41] Cuschieri A, Jakimowicz JJ, van Spreeuwel J. Laparoscopic distal 70% pancreatectomy and splenectomy for chronic pancreatitis. Ann Surg. 1996; 223:280–5.

[42] Wolfgang CL, Herman JM, Laheru DA, Klein AP, Erdek MA, Fishman EK, et al. Recent progress in pancreatic cancer. CA Cancer J Clin. 2013; 63(5):318–48.

[43] Kleeff J, Diener MK, Z'graggen K, Hinz U, Wagner M, Bachmann J, et al. Distal pancreatectomy: risk factors for surgical failure in 302 consecutive cases. Ann Surg. 2007; 245(4):573–82.

[44] Lillemoe KD, Kaushal S, Cameron JL, Sohn TA, Pitt HA, Yeo CJ. Distal pancreatectomy: indications and outcomes in 235 patients. Ann Surg. 1999; 229(5): 693–8.

[45] Adam MA, Choudhury K, Goffredo P, Reed SD, Blazer D 3rd, Roman SA, et al. Minimally invasive distal pancreatectomy for cancer: short-term oncologic outcomes in 1733 patients. World J Surg. 2015; 39(10):2564–72.

[46] Braga M, Pecorelli N, Ferrari D, Balzano G, Zuliani W, Castoldi R. Results of 100 consecutive laparoscopic distal pancreatectomies: postoperative outcome, cost-benefit analysis, and quality of life assessment. Surg Endosc. 2015; 29(7):1871–8.

[47] Daouadi M, Zureikat AH, Zenati MS, Choudry H, Tsung A, Bartlett DL, et al. Robot-assisted minimally invasive distal pancreatectomy is superior to the laparoscopic technique. Ann Surg. 2013; 257(1):128–32.

[48] DiNorcia J, Schrope Ba., Lee MK, Reavey PL, Rosen SJ, Lee J a., et al. Laparoscopic distal pancreatectomy offers shorter hospital stays with fewer complications. J Gastrointest Surg. 2010; 14(11):1804–12.

[49] Gumbs AA, Croner R, Rodriguez A, Zuker N, Perrakis A, Gayet B. 200 Consecutive laparoscopic pancreatic resections performed with a robotically controlled laparoscope holder. Surg Endosc. 2013; 27(10): 3781–91.

[50] Jayaraman S, Gonen M, Brennan MF, D'Angelica MI, DeMatteo RP, Fong Y, et al. Laparoscopic distal pancreatectomy: evolution of a technique at a single institution. J Am Coll Surg. 2010; 211(4):503–9.

[51] Jean-Philippe A, Alexandre J, Christophe L, Denis C, Masson B, Fernández-Cruz L, et al. Laparoscopic spleen-preserving distal pancreatectomy. JAMA Surg. 2013; 148(3): 246–52.

[52] Kneuertz PJ, Patel SH, Chu CK, Fisher SB, Maithel SK, Sarmiento JM, et al. Laparoscopic distal pancreatectomy: Trends and lessons learned through an 11-year experience. J Am Coll Surg. 2012; 215(2):167–76.

[53] Lee SY, Allen PJ, Sadot E, D'Angelica MI, DeMatteo RP, Fong Y, et al. Distal pancreatectomy: A single institution's experience in open, laparoscopic, and robotic approaches. J Am Coll Surg. 2015; 220(1):18–27.

[54] Malleo G, Damoli I, Marchegiani G, Esposito A, Marchese T, Salvia R, et al. Laparoscopic distal pancreatectomy: Analysis of trends in surgical techniques, patient selection, and outcomes. Surg Endosc. 2015; 29(7):1952–62.

[55] Mendoza AS 3rd, Han HS, Ahn S, Yoon YS, Cho JY, Choi Y. Predictive factors associated with postoperative pancreatic fistula after laparoscopic distal pancreatectomy: A 10-year single-institution experience. Surg Endosc. 2016; 30(2): 649–56.

[56] Nakamura M, Wakabayashi G, Miyasaka Y, Tanaka M, Morikawa T, Unno M, et al. Multicenter comparative study of laparoscopic and open distal pancreatectomy using propensity score-matching. J Hepatobiliary Pancreat Sci. 2015; 22(10):731–6.

[57] Rutz DR, Squires MH, Maithel SK, Sarmiento JM, Etra JW, Perez SD, et al. Cost comparison analysis of open versus laparoscopic distal pancreatectomy. HPB. 2014; 16(10):907–14.

[58] Sahakyan MA, Kazaryan AM, Rawashdeh M, Fuks D, Shmavonyan M, Haugvik SP, et al. Laparoscopic distal pancreatectomy for pancreatic ductal adenocarcinoma: Results of a multicenter cohort study on 196 patients. Surg Endosc. 2015 [Epub ahead of print]

[59] Sharpe SM, Talamonti MS, Wang E, Bentrem DJ, Roggin KK, Prinz RA, et al. The laparoscopic approach to distal pancreatectomy for ductal adenocarcinoma results in shorter lengths of stay without compromising oncologic outcomes. Am J Surg. 2015; 209:557–563

[60] Shin SH, Kim SC, Song KB, Hwang DW, Lee JH, Lee D, et al. A Comparative Study of laparoscopic vs open distal pancreatectomy for left-sided ductal adenocarcinoma: A propensity score-matched analysis. J Am Coll Surg. 2015; 220(2):177–85.

[61] Song KB, Kim SC, Park JB, Kim YH, Jung YS, Kim MH, et al. Single-center experience of laparoscopic left pancreatic resection in 359 consecutive patients: Changing the surgical paradigm of left pancreatic resection. Surg Endosc Other Interv Tech. 2011; 25:3364–72.

[62] Stauffer JA, Rosales-Velderrain A, Goldberg RF, Bowers SP, Asbun HJ. Comparison of open with laparoscopic distal pancreatectomy: A single institution's transition over a 7-year period. HPB. 2013; 15(2):149–55.

[63] Vijan SS. Laparoscopic vs open distal pancreatectomy. Arch Surg. 2010; 145(7):616–21.

[64] Xourafas D, Tavakkoli A, Clancy TE, Ashley SW. Distal pancreatic resection for neuroendocrine tumors: Is laparoscopic really better than open? J Gastrointest Surg. 2015; 19(5):831–40.

[65] Yan J, Kuang T, Ji D, Xu X, Wang D, Zhang R, et al. Laparoscopic versus open distal pancreatectomy for benign or premalignant pancreatic neoplasms: A two-center comparative study. J Zhejiang Univ Sci B. 2015; 16(7):573–9.

[66] Yoon Y-S, Lee KH, Han H-S, Cho JY, Jang JY, Kim S-W, et al. Effects of laparoscopic versus open surgery on splenic vessel patency after spleen and splenic vessel-preserving distal pancreatectomy: A retrospective multicenter study. Surg Endosc. 2015; 29(3): 583–8.

[67] Zhou ZQ, Kim SC, Song KB, Park K-M, Lee JH, Lee Y-J. Laparoscopic spleen-preserving distal pancreatectomy: Comparative study of spleen preservation with splenic vessel resection and splenic vessel preservation. World J Surg. 2014; 38(11):2973–9.

[68] Ricci C, Casadei R, Buscemi S, Taffurelli G, D'Ambra M, Pacilio CA, et al. Laparoscopic distal pancreatectomy: What factors are related to the learning curve? Surg Today. 2015; 45(1): 50–6.

[69] Braga M, Ridolfi C, Balzano G, Castoldi R, Pecorelli N, Di Carlo V. Learning curve for laparoscopic distal pancreatectomy in a high-volume hospital. Updates Surg. 2012; 64:179–83

[70] Goyal K, Einstein D, Ibarra RA, Yao M, Kunos C, Ellis R, Brindle J, et al. Stereotactic body radiation therapy for nonresectable tumors of the pancreas. J Surg Res. 2012; 174(2): 319–25.

[71] Barbaros U, Sümer A, Demirel T, Karakullukçu N, Batman B, Içscan Y, et al. Single incision laparoscopic pancreas resection for pancreatic metastasis of renal cell carcinoma. JSLS. 2010; 14(4):566–70.

[72] Bracale U, Lazzara F, Andreuccetti J, Stabilini C, Pignata G. Single-access laparoscopic subtotal spleno-pancreatectomy for pancreatic adenocarcinoma. Minim Invasive Ther Allied Technol. 2014; 23(2):106–9.

[73] Chang SKY, Lomanto D, Mayasari M. Single-port laparoscopic spleen preserving distal pancreatectomy. Minim Invasive Surg. 2012; 2012:1–4.

[74] Han HJ, Yoon SY, Song TJ, Choi SB, Kim WB, Choi SY, Park SH. Single-port laparoscopic distal pancreatectomy: Initial experience. J Laparoendosc Adv Surg Tech A. 2014; 24(12): 858–63.

[75] Haugvik SP, Røsok BI, Waage A, Mathisen O, Edwin B. Single-incision versus conventional laparoscopic distal pancreatectomy: A single-institution case-control study. Langenbecks Arch Surg. 2013; 398:1091–6.

[76] Misawa T, Ito R, Futagawa Y, Fujiwara Y, Kitamura H, Tsutsui N, et al. Single-incision laparoscopic distal pancreatectomy with or without splenic preservation: How we do it. Asian J Endosc Surg. 2012; 5(4):195–9.

[77] Srikanth G, Shetty N, Dubey D. Single incision laparoscopic distal pancreatectomy with splenectomy for neuroendocrine tumor of the tail of pancreas. J Minim Access Surg. 2013; 9(3):132–5.

[78] Giulianotti PC, Coratti A, Angelini M, Sabrana F, Cecconi S, Balestracci T, Caravaglios G. Robotics in general surgery. Arch Surg. 2003; 138:777–84.

[79] Polanco PM, Zenati MS, Hogg ME, Shakir M, Boone BA, Bartlett DL, et al. An analysis of risk factors for pancreatic fistula after robotic pancreaticoduodenectomy: outcomes from a consecutive series of standardized pancreatic reconstructions. Surg Endosc. 2016;30(4):1523–9.

[80] Boone Ba, Zenati M, Hogg ME, Steve J, Moser AJ, Bartlett DL, et al. Assessment of quality outcomes for robotic pancreaticoduodenectomy: Identification of the learning curve. JAMA Surg. 2015; 15232(5):1–7.

[81] Hanna EM, Rozario N, Rupp C, Sindram D, Iannitti DA, Martinie JB. Robotic hepato-biliary and pancreatic surgery: Lessons learned and predictors for conversion. Int J Med Robot Comput Assist Surg. 2013; 9(2): 152–9.

[82] Shakir M, Boone Ba, Polanco PM, Zenati MS, Hogg ME, Tsung A, et al. The learning curve for robotic distal pancreatectomy: An analysis of outcomes of the first 100 consecutive cases at a high-volume pancreatic centre. HPB. 2015; 17(7): 580–6.

[83] Napoli N, Kauffmann EF, Perrone VG, Miccoli M, Brozzetti S, Boggi U. The learning curve in robotic distal pancreatectomy. Updates Surg. 2015; 67(3): 257–64.

[84] Chen S, Chen J-Z, Zhan Q, Deng X-X, Shen B-Y, Peng C-H, et al. Robot-assisted laparoscopic versus open pancreaticoduodenectomy: A prospective, matched, mid-term follow-up study. Surg Endosc. 2015; 29(12):3698–711.

[85] Giulianotti PC, Sbrana F, Bianco FM, Elli EF, Shah G, Addeo P, et al. Robot-assisted laparoscopic pancreatic surgery: Single-surgeon experience. Surg Endosc. 2010; 24(7): 1646–57.

[86] Zeh HJ, Zureikat AH, Secrest A, Dauoudi M, Bartlett D, Moser AJ. Outcomes after robot-assisted pancreaticoduodenectomy for periampullary lesions. Ann Surg Oncol. 2012; 19(3): 864–70.

[87] Zureikat AH, Moser AJ, Boone BA, Bartlett DL, Zenati M, Zeh HJ 3rd. 250 robotic pancreatic resections: Safety and feasibility. Ann Surg. 2013; 258(4):554–9.

[88] Chen S, Zhan Q, Chen J, Jin J-B, Deng X-X, Chen H, et al. Robotic approach improves spleen-preserving rate and shortens postoperative hospital stay of laparoscopic distal pancreatectomy: A matched cohort study. Surg Endosc. 2015; 29(12):3507–18.

[89] Cleary K, Wilson E, Ordas S, Banovac F. Navigation. In: Jolesz FA, editor. Intraoperative Imaging and Image-Guided Therapy. Springer, New York. 2014.

[90] Langø T, Vijayan S, Rethy A, Våpenstad C, Solberg OV, Mårvik R, et al. Navigated laparoscopic ultrasound in abdominal soft tissue surgery: Technological overview and perspectives. Int J Comput Assist Radiol Surg. 2012; 7(4):585–99.

[91] Askeland C, Solberg OV, Bakeng JBL, Reinertsen I, Tangen GA, Hofstad EF, et al. CustusX: An open-source research platform for image-guided therapy. Int J Comput Assist Radiol Surg. 2016; 11: 505–19.

[92] Sánchez-Margallo FM, Sánchez-Margallo JA. Computer-assisted minimally invasive surgery: Image-guided interventions and robotic surgery. In: Xiaojun C, editor. Computer-Assisted Surgery: New Developments, Applications and Potential Hazards. New York: Nova Science Publishers. 2015. pp. 43–95.

[93] Li W, An L, Liu R, Yao K, Hu M, Zhao G, et al. Laparoscopic ultrasound enhances diagnosis and localization of insulinoma in pancreatic head and neck for laparoscopic surgery with satisfactory postsurgical outcomes. Ultrasound Med Biol. 2011; 37(7): 1017–23.

[94] Våpenstad C, Rethy A, Langø T, Selbekk T, Ystgaard B, Hernes TAN, et al. Laparoscopic ultrasound: A survey of its current and future use, requirements, and integration with navigation technology. Surg Endosc. 2010; 24(12):2944–53.

[95] Piccolboni D, Ciccone F, Settembre a, Corcione F. Laparoscopic intra-operative ultrasound in liver and pancreas resection: Analysis of 93 cases. J Ultrasound. 2010; 13(1): 3–8.

[96] Barabino M, Santambrogio R, Pisani Ceretti A, Scalzone R, Montorsi M, Opocher E. Is there still a role for laparoscopy combined with laparoscopic ultrasonography in the staging of pancreatic cancer? Surg Endosc. 2011; 25(1):160–5.

[97] Fernández-Cruz L, Sáenz A, Astudillo E, Martinez I, Hoyos S, Pantoja JP, et al. Outcome of laparoscopic pancreatic surgery: Endocrine and nonendocrine tumors. World J Surg. 2002; 26(8):1057–65.

[98] Schachter PP, Shimonov M, Czerniak A. The role of laparoscopy and laparoscopic ultrasound in the diagnosis of cystic lesions of the pancreas. Gastrointest Endosc Clin N Am. 2002; 12(4):759–67.

[99] Schwarz L, Fleming J, Katz M, Lee J, Aloia T, Vauthey N, Conrad C. Total laparoscopic central pancreatectomy with pancreaticogastrostomy for high-risk cystic neoplasm. Ann Surg Oncol. 2016; 23(3): 1035.

[100] Catheline JM, Turner R, Rizk N, Barrat C, Champault G The use of diagnostic laparoscopy supported by laparoscopic ultrasonography in the assessment of pancreatic cancer. Surg Endosc. 1999; 13(3):239–45.

[101] Chance B. Near-infrared images using continuous, phase-modulated, and pulsed light with quantitation of blood and blood oxygenation. Ann N Y Acad Sci. 1998; 838: 29–45.

[102] Vahrmeijer AL, Hutteman M, van der Vorst JR, van de Velde CJH, Frangioni JV. Image-guided cancer surgery using near-infrared fluorescence. Nat Rev Clin Oncol. 2013; 10(9):507–18.

[103] Winer JH, Choi HS, Gibbs-Strauss SL, Ashitate Y, Colson YL, Frangioni JV. Intraoperative localization of insulinoma and normal pancreas using invisible near-infrared fluorescent light. Ann Surg Oncol. 2010; 17(4):1094–100.

[104] Chi C, Du Y, Ye J, Kou D, Qiu J, Wang J, et al. Intraoperative imaging-guided cancer surgery: From current fluorescence molecular imaging methods to future multi-modality imaging technology. Theranostics. 2014; 4(11):1072–84.

[105] Yokoyama N, Otani T, Hashidate H, Maeda C, Katada T, Sudo N. et al. Real-time detection of hepatic micrometastases from pancreatic cancer by intraoperative fluorescence imaging: Preliminary results of a prospective study. Cancer. 2012; 118:2813–9.

[106] Van der Vorst JR, Vahrmeijer AL, Hutteman M. Near-infrared fluorescence imaging of a solitary fibrous tumor of the pancreas using methylene blue. World J Gastrointest Surg. 2012; 4(7):180–4.

[107] Verbeek FPR, van der Vorst JR, Schaafsma BE, Hutteman M, Bonsing BA, van Leeuwen FWB, et al. Image-guided hepatopancreatobiliary surgery using near-infrared fluorescent light. J Hepatobiliary Pancreat Sci. 2012; 19(6):626–37.

[108] Subar D, Pietrasz D, Fuks D, Gayet B. A novel technique for reducing pancreatic fistulas after pancreaticojejunostomy. J Surg Case Rep. 2015; 2015(7): rjv074.

[109] Metildi CA, Kaushal S, Luiken GA, et al. Advantages of fluorescence-guided laparoscopic surgery of pancreatic cancer labeled with fluorescent anti-carcinoembryonic antigen antibodies in an orthotopic mouse model. J Am Coll Surg. 2014;219:132–41.

[110] Sorger H, Hofstad EF, Amundsen T, Langø T, Leira HO. A novel platform for electromagnetic navigated ultrasound bronchoscopy (EBUS). Int J Comput Assist Radiol Surg. 2015 [Epub ahead of print].

[111] Manstad-Hulaas F, Tangen GA, Dahl T, Hernes TA, Aadahl P. Three-dimensional electromagnetic navigation vs. fluoroscopy for endovascular aneurysm repair: a prospective feasibility study in patients. J Endovasc Ther. 2012; 19(1):70–8.

[112] Langø T, Tangen GA, Mårvik R, Ystgaard B, Yavuz Y, Kaspersen JH, et al. Navigation in laparoscopy-prototype research platform for improved image-guided surgery. Minim Invasive Ther Allied Technol. 2008; 17(1):17–33.

[113] Bø LE, Hofstad EF, Lindseth F, Hernes TA. Versatile robotic probe calibration for position tracking in ultrasound imaging. Phys Med Biol. 2015; 60(9): 3499–513.

[114] Sugimoto M, Yasuda H, Koda K, Suzuki M, Yamazaki M, Tezuka T, et al. Image overlay navigation by markerless surface registration in gastrointestinal, hepatobiliary and pancreatic surgery. J Hepatobiliary Pancreat Sci. 2010; 17(5):629–36.

Chapter 4

Laparoscopic Left Adrenalectomy with Submesocolic and Retropancreatic Approach

Andrea Balla, Silvia Quaresima, Ardit Seitaj,
Andrea M. Isidori, Franco Iafrate and
Alessandro M. Paganini

Additional information is available at the end of the chapter

http://dx.doi.org/10.5772/66457

Abstract

Introduction: The safety and efficacy of laparoscopic transperitoneal lateral adrenalectomy and retroperitoneoscopic adrenalectomy have been reported. The aim is to report the authors' experience in laparoscopic left adrenalectomy with an alternative transperitoneal submesocolic and retropancreatic approach with patient supine.

Research methods: The authors have performed laparoscopic transperitoneal submesocolic, retropancreatic adrenalectomy for both benign and malignant, functioning lesions >4 cm in diameter or with smaller lesions but having an imaging pattern suspicious of malignancy or of sub-clinically secreting tumors. After opening the posterior peritoneum at the root of the transverse mesocolon and Gerota's fascia, the junction of the inferior adrenal vein with the left renal vein is identified. The adrenal vein is then prepared and divided, followed by mobilization and removal of the left adrenal gland.

Conclusion: Early ligation of the adrenal vein is the most relevant technical feature of this procedure to avoid the release of catecholamines, hormones or neoplastic cells which could occur during manipulation of the gland prior to ligation of the main adrenal vein. Moreover, this approach makes it possible to perform associated procedures, including a bilateral adrenalectomy, without the need to reposition the patient on the operative table, but simply by positioning additional trocars.

Keywords: adrenal tumors, laparoscopic adrenalectomy, pheochromocytoma, transperitoneal anterior approach, submesocolic retropancreatic approach

1. Introduction

The surgical approach to the adrenal gland has raised debate among surgeons due to its retroperitoneal location and for the complexity in the management of secreting tumors, particularly in case of pheochromocytoma (PHE) [1–3]. Traditionally, open adrenalectomy is made difficult due to its deep anatomical location, and it is associated with up to 39% morbidity rate and prolonged hospital stay [1–3]. In 1992, Gagner described the first laparoscopic adrenalectomy (LA) by a transperitoneal approach with the patient in the lateral decubitus position [4, 5]. This initial experience has been followed by others using the same approach or, alternatively, the retroperitoneal approach with the patient in the prone or in the lateral decubitus position [6, 7] and the transperitoneal approach with the patient supine [8]. Several reports have confirmed the safety and efficacy of these techniques, and minimally, invasive adrenalectomy is presently considered the treatment of choice for a variety of benign lesions, including lesions of the medulla [9, 10].

The aim of the present chapter is to report the authors' experience with left laparoscopic adrenalectomy (LA) using an original transperitoneal submesocolic and retropancreatic approach with patient supine, to describe the patient's preparation for surgery as well as the operative details of this procedure.

2. Methods

In order to establish the diagnosis in case of adrenal secreting lesions, all patients undergo complete hormonal evaluation as previously reported [11]. Diurnal serum cortisol, dehydroepiandrosterone (DHEAS), plasma adrenocorticotropic hormone (ACTH), testosterone, androstenedione, urinary free cortisol (UFC), 17-hydroxyprogesterone (17-OHP), renin activity, aldosterone and urinary catecholamine levels are measured, together with overnight 1 mg dexamethasone suppression test (DST) [11]. Aldosterone-producing adenoma, pheochromocytoma and Cushing's syndrome are diagnosed on the basis of high plasma aldosterone, plasma renin activity (PRA) ratio (>40) and unsuppressed aldosterone after sodium load, elevated urinary metanephrines, elevated UFC, abnormal serum cortisol, inadequate cortisol suppression after 1-mg dexamethasone and low and/or suppressed plasma ACTH [11]. When no specific signs and/or symptoms of autonomous hormone secretion are present, or abnormal hypothalamus-pituitary-adrenal axis tests and radiological imaging suggesting the presence of an adrenocortical lesion, a diagnosis of nonfunctioning adenoma is made [11].

All patients are studied with computed tomography (CT) scan and magnetic resonance imaging (MRI). An attenuation value of 1O or less Hounsfield units (HU) on unenhanced CT scan is suggestive for the presence of a benign adrenocortical adenoma [12]. Relative contrast washout of >40% and an absolute contrast washout of >60% are suggestive for an adenoma, with 92% specificity and 98% sensitivity rates, respectively [13, 14]. In all sequences during MRI,

adrenocortical adenomas are homogeneous, with mild gadolinium enhancement [12], with low or equal signal intensity as the liver on T2-weighted images may appear on lower signal intensity than the rest of the adrenal gland [12]. Chemical shift imaging can be done during MRI to identify fat within the lesion as decreased signal intensity relative to normal tissue [12]. For carcinomas, the attenuation on unenhanced studies is higher than 10HU on CT scan [15]. On contrast-enhanced studies, carcinomas enhance greedily due to their vascularity, and the enhancement pattern may be homogeneous, unless there is central necrosis [15, 16]. The relative percentage washout of carcinomas is <40% [17]. At MRI, adrenal carcinomas are noted for heterogeneity on T1-weighted images, with intermediate to high signal intensity [18]. Heterogeneity is also noted on T2-weighted images due to hemorrhage and/or necrosis [18]. Based on these criteria, adrenal lesions larger than 4cm in diameter or with smaller but having an imaging pattern suspicious of malignancy or of sub-clinically secreting tumors are an indication for laparoscopic adrenalectomy.

2.1. Patient's preoperative preparation

2.1.1. Pheochromocytoma

Alpha-blockers (doxazosin 20mg/day), starting at least 15days before surgery, are administered. If patients reported episodes of tachycardia, beta-blockers are also administered (atenolol 100–200mg/day orally). On the day before surgery, treatment with alpha-blockers is discontinued, and intravenous (iv) normal saline 2000cc is administered to expand the plasma volume [19].

2.1.2. Conn's syndrome

Iv hydrocortisone 100mg is administered at induction of anesthesia. Iv spironolactone is used for potassium control [20].

2.1.3. Cushing's syndrome

Iv hydrocortisone 100mg is administered at induction of anesthesia and then iv hydrocortisone 50mg every 8h [20].

2.2. Surgical technique

2.2.1. Left adrenalectomy: transperitoneal anterior submesocolic and retropancreatic approach

Surgery is performed under general anesthesia. An orogastric tube and urinary catheter are positioned. Intraoperative patients' monitoring includes intra-arterial radial artery catheter for continuous blood pressure measurement and a central venous catheter (subclavian or internal jugular access) for rapid infusion of liquids. Pneumoperitoneum is usually established with a Veress needle at the umbilicus or with an open technique and Hasson cannula, in case of the presence of abdominal scars from previous surgery. Pneumoperitoneum is set at a pressure of 12–13mmHg, with carbon dioxide flow adjusted at 30lt/min. Four trocars and a 30°/45°

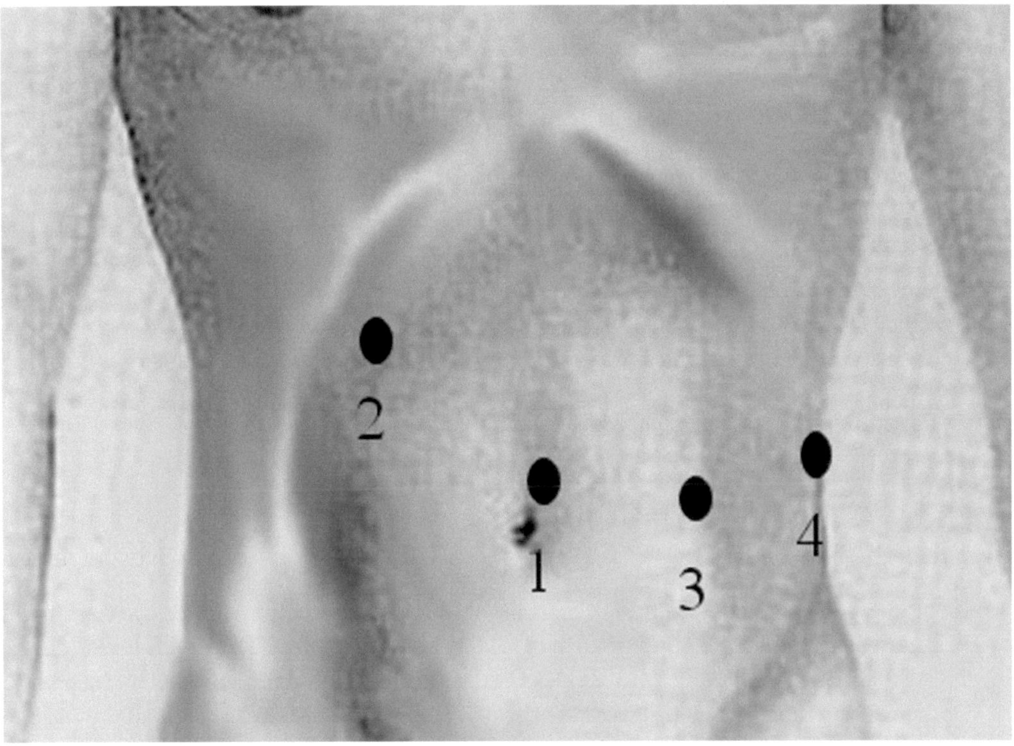

Figure 1. Trocars' position during left transperitoneal submesocolic and retropancreatic adrenalectomy. The surgeon and first assistant stand on the left of the patient, while the second assistant stands on the right.

forward oblique optic are used. This approach is performed with the patient supine, in slight anti-Trendelenburg position and with the operating table turned 30° with the side opposite the lesion down, to facilitate exposure of the surgical field. The surgeon stands on the side which is ipsilateral to the lesion.

After induction of pneumoperitoneum, the first 12-mm optical trocar (n. 1) is inserted on the left of the midline above the umbilicus (**Figure 1**). A second 12-mm trocar (n. 2) is inserted under vision on the right midclavicular line below the right costal arch. The third and fourth 12-mm trocars are placed one on the left midclavicular line along with the transverse umbilical line (n. 3) and other on the left anterior axillary line (n. 4), respectively (**Figure 1**). The 10-mm laparoscope is introduced from trocar (n. 3), while trocars 1 and 4 are the operating ones. With atraumatic forceps introduced from trocar (n. 2), the transverse mesocolon is raised by the assistant. This maneuver discloses the first jejunal loop at the ligament of Treitz, and it shows the arch of the inferior mesenteric vein. The operative table is tilted with the left side of the patient up, which allows the surgeon to displace the first jejunal loops on the patient's right side (**Figure 2**). The posterior peritoneum is opened at the insertion of the transverse mesocolon and posteriorly to the lower edge of the pancreas, between the first jejunal loop and the arch of the inferior mesenteric vein or immediately lateral to this vessel, according to

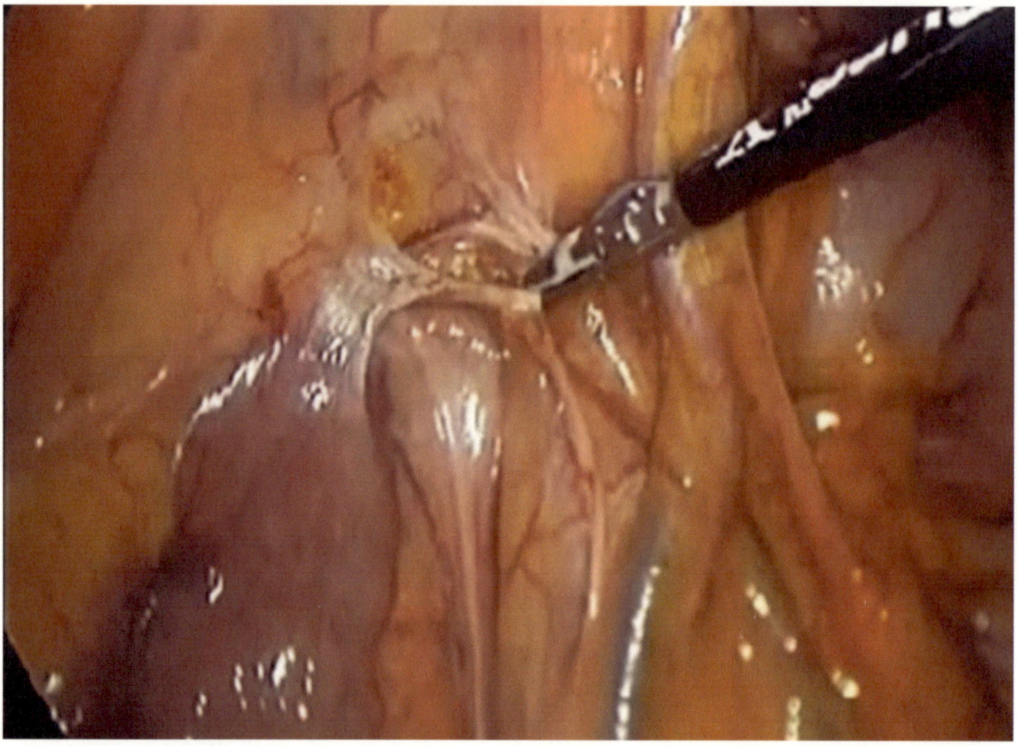

Figure 2. After raising the transverse mesocolon and displacing the first jejunal loop on the patient's right side, the posterior peritoneum is divided close to the arch of the inferior mesenteric vein.

its distance from the jejunum. Toldt's fascia appears at this point as a whitish film. The dissection then proceeds posteriorly along the retro-pancreatic space, after raising the body of the pancreas with an atraumatic instrument held by the surgeon's left hand. The splenic vein is visible at this point running along the posterior aspect of the pancreas. Gerota's fascia is now opened to visualize the left renal vein, which is followed medially, until the left inferior adrenal vein is identified. This is cautiously prepared and divided between clips (AcuClip, Tyco/Healtcare, Norwalk, Connecticut, USA, **Figure 3**). No manipulation of the left adrenal gland has yet occurred prior to division of the adrenal vein because the gland is located cranially to this vessel. Only at this point, the gland is mobilized using a radiofrequency (LigaSure™ tissue fusion, Covidien, Mansfield, Massachusetts, USA) or ultrasonic (Ultracision, Harmonic Scalpel, Ethicon Endo Surgery, Cincinnati, Ohio, USA) device, and the specimen is removed from the abdominal cavity inside a specimen retrieval bag after slightly enlarging the periumbilical trocar incision [19].

Near-infrared indocyanine green (NIR-ICG) fluorescence may be employed during surgery and may be useful to aid in vascular structures and adrenal gland identification amidst retroperitoneal and perirenal fat, particularly in obese patients, to improve the safety of laparoscopic adrenalectomy.

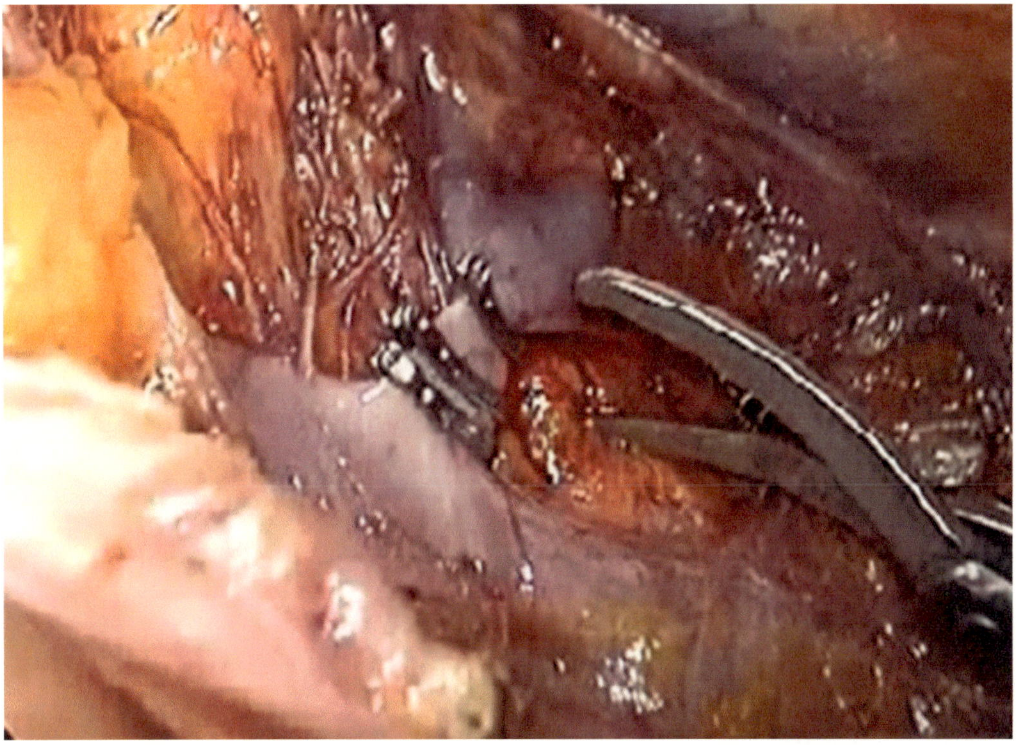

Figure 3. The left adrenal vein is divided between clips. Confluence of the diaphragmatic vein to the left adrenal vein is visible.

3. Discussion

Surgery is the standard treatment of Conn's syndrome, Cushing's disease, pheochromocytoma, primary adrenal cancer and adrenal metastases. After the introduction of minimally invasive adrenalectomy, this has now become the treatment of choice [8, 21–26]. Minimally, invasive adrenalectomy is mostly performed either with a transperitoneal lateral approach or with a retroperitoneal approach [4]. The laparoscopic transperitoneal anterior approach has been proposed only by few centers [8, 11, 19, 23, 24, 26].

The transperitoneal lateral approach, originally described by Gagner et al. [4], is performed with the patient in the lateral decubitus position. It gives excellent exposure of the operative field with a wide working space, and it facilitates orientation by providing readily identifiable anatomical landmarks [27]. Its proponents report several advantages, such as a rapid and direct access to the gland without the need to retract any organ and with minimal patient trauma [28], a clear operative field due to gravity that keeps blood and bowel away from it and the need for less surgical dissection on the left side, as compared to the anterior approach [26]. By the authors' opinion, the main disadvantage of the lateral approach is that it does not provide early ligation of the adrenal vein prior to gland manipulation, which the authors

believe to be important so as to avoid pressure instability in case of secreting adenomas, and particularly of pheochromocytoma, and which would also be oncologically correct [11, 19, 29].

Retroperitoneal adrenalectomy (RA) has also been reported to be safe and effective [21, 30, 31]. According to its proponents, it is preferred to reduce the risks and possible complications of a transperitoneal access, such as incisional hernias and paralytic ileus from bowel manipulation [4, 7]. It has been reported to require less analgesics due to lower postoperative pain [27] and to be associated with earlier recovery of bowel function, possibly leading to shorter hospital stay [27]. However, minimal postoperative pain, early liquid diet and a short hospital stay have been reported also after a laparoscopic approach [5, 6, 26, 27]. RA is preferred in patients with abdominal adhesions from previous surgery and in obese patients [32]. Moreover, several authors reported a shorter operative time [28]. According to Walz et al. [33], a 7 cm hormonally active tumor or a 4–7 cm nonfunctioning tumor may be indications for a retroperitoneal approach. By the opinion of these authors, severe obesity, simultaneous abdominal pathology, patients with evident signs of malignancy or a tumor exceeding 8 cm are contraindications for the retroperitoneal approach [33]. In our opinion, the patient's position during RA is unfavorable for rapid conversion to open surgery in case of major bleeding and may itself impair or worsen the hemodynamic conditions of the patient [8].

Moreover, both lateral LA and RA do not allow to perform associated surgical procedures [11, 19, 34]. In lateral LA, exploration of the contralateral gland is not possible without repositioning the patient [11, 19, 34], which increases the operative time.

To reduce the risk of catecholamines, hormones or neoplastic cells spread from the adrenal gland, the authors introduced the laparoscopic transperitoneal submesocolic and retropancreatic approach with the patient supine. This approach was originally described by Pierre Delbet in 1912 [35]. Its main advantages are the limited extent of the dissection and early identification, ligation and division of the left adrenal vein which is obtained prior to any gland manipulation. This aspect is particularly important in case of secreting lesions. In fact, the authors consider early clipping of the main adrenal vein to be of upmost importance, together with avoiding any manipulation of the gland prior to adrenal vein ligation [11, 19, 24, 26, 36].

With respect to the transperitoneal anterior and lateral approaches, it does not require mobilization of the left colonic flexure or of the spleno-pancreatic complex to gain access to the adrenal gland, with reduction of the operative time and of potential operative risks. However, it does require experience in advanced laparoscopic surgery because the operation is conducted in a restricted working space adjacent to major venous vessels, such as the left renal and splenic veins, and the aorta [11, 19, 37].

In case of LA or RA for pheochromocytoma, because of the complexity of the disease, the operation should be performed only in centers with a well established, multidisciplinary experience in the diagnosis and treatment of adrenal gland pathology. In fact, surgery for pheochromocytoma is at risk of hypotensive or hypertensive crisis, or both, due to an excess in catecholamine release, which cannot be completely prevented even by adequate preoperative preparation with α-blockers [10]. The aim of medical treatment prior to surgery is not the

reduction of hormonal secretion but the prevention of the peripheral effects of catecholamines secreted by the tumor, so that the patient may undergo surgery under the best cardiovascular conditions [38]. Advances in intraoperative monitoring and the introduction of preoperative α1-receptors' blockade have radically reduced the mortality rate [39]. A significant increase in the rates of plasma norepinephrine release related to mobilization of the adrenal gland has been reported during LA with a lateral approach [39]. One study also reported that severe hypertension was triggered by direct manipulation of the adrenal gland [10]. Instead, no significant intraoperative change in blood pressure was observed following this surgical strategy in case of pheochromocytoma [19]. Based on the authors' data, the anterior laparoscopic submesocolic and retropancreatic approach for treatment of secreting adrenal lesions is safe [11, 19, 24].

Authors	*N*	**Approach**	**Mean age (years)**	**Mean oper. time (min.)**	**Conversion (%)**	**Morbidity (%)**	**H.S. (days)**
Hazzan [2]	24	Lateral	45.4	188	7	16	4
Vargas [3]	20	Lateral	47	193	10	10	3.1
Gagner [5]	100	Lateral	46	130	3	12	2.5
Bonjer [6]	79	RP	50	114	6.3	10.1	2
Salomon [7]	21	RP	46	116	0	19	3.4
Lang [9]	56	RP	36.2	52	1.8	1.7	5.2
Janetschek [10]	19	Lateral	49.7	150	0	16	7
Mohammadi-Fallah [27]	11	Lateral	43	129	0	9.1	3.6
	12	RP	42	128	8.3	8.3	3.1
Dickson [30]	23	Lateral	42	145	4.3	8.7	3.1
	23	RP	47	100	13	13	1.9
Fernández-Cruz [31]	16	Lateral	36	89	12.5	12.5	3
	14	RP	47	105	14.2	0	2.75
Walz [33]	560	RP	49.2	67	1.7	11.8	–
Cabalag [44]	13	Lateral	47	105	0	30.7	2
	10	RP	61	90	0	10	1
Paganini [11]	19	LASA	54	92	0	0	4.4
Paganini [19]	37	LASA	54	82.7	0	0	3.85
Matsuda [29]	75	Anterior	–	221	0	3.9	10.2
Linos [45]	18	Anterior	48.7	116	5.5	0	2.3

N, number of patients; H.S, hospital stay; RP, retroperitoneal; LASA, left anterior submesocolic approach.

Table 1. Patient series reported in the literature.

http://dx.doi.org/10.5772/66457

Some authors [40, 41] consider tumors larger than 6cm to be a contraindication for a minimally invasive approach, due to the risk of malignancy. In the authors' experience, the size of the largest lesion up to 10cm in diameter did not affect the feasibility and the outcome of the procedure or the operative time [11, 19, 24]. This observation has been confirmed by Parnaby et al. [42], whose results are in agreement with the authors' experience [11, 19, 24].

Moreover, the supine position of the patient allows one to perform associated diagnostic [43] or operative procedures, such as contralateral adrenalectomy, without the need to reposition the patient on the operative table. In the authors' experience, the submesocolic approach was associated with a significant reduction in the operative time, as compared to the laparoscopic traditional anterior approach, which compares favorably also with the operative time of the lateral and retroperitoneal approaches reported in the literature (**Table 1**) [2, 3, 5–7, 9–11, 19, 27, 29–31, 33, 44, 45].

Independently from the approach that is followed, the recent introduction of a dedicated laparoscopic instrumentation to detect near-infrared fluorescence with indocyanine green (NIR-ICG) improves visualization of the inferior adrenal vein and of the adrenal gland with respect to the surrounding fat, making their identification easier [46, 47]. In the authors' opinion, this instrumentation might improve the safety of the procedure, as well as the oncological outcome in case of adrenal cancer or metastases.

LA with transperitoneal submesocolic and retropancreatic approach has proven to be safe and effective [11, 19, 24], and its results are in line with those reported in the most recent literature [48] after RA and lateral LA. Early ligation of the adrenal vein is the most important technical feature of this technique in every type of lesion. For more objective results, a multicenter randomized clinical trial comparing the submesocolic approach with lateral LA and RA for left adrenalectomy would be required.

Author details

Andrea Balla[1]*, Silvia Quaresima[1], Ardit Seitaj[1], Andrea M. Isidori[2], Franco Iafrate[3] and Alessandro M. Paganini[1]*

*Address all correspondence to: andrea.balla@gmail.com and alessandro.paganini@uniroma1.it

1 Department of General Surgery and Surgical Specialties "Paride Stefanini", Sapienza University of Rome, Rome, Italy

2 Department of Experimental Medicine, Sapienza University of Rome, Rome, Italy

3 Department of Radiological Oncological and Pathological Sciences, Sapienza University of Rome, Rome, Italy

References

[1] Wang HS, Li CC, Chou YH, Wang CJ, Wu WJ, Huang CH. Comparison of laparoscopic adrenalectomy with open surgery for adrenal tumors. Kaohsiung J Med Sci. 2009 Aug;25 (8):438–44. doi:10.1016/S1607-551X(09)70539-X

[2] Hazzan D, Shiloni E, Golijanin D, Jurim O, Gross D, Reissman P. Laparoscopic vs open adrenalectomy for benign adrenal neoplasm. Surg Endosc. 2001 Nov;15(11):1356–8.

[3] Vargas HI, Kavoussi LR, Bartlett DL, Wagner JR, Venzon DJ, Fraker DL, Alexander HR, Linehan WM, Walther MM. Laparoscopic adrenalectomy: a new standard of care. Urology. 1997 May;49(5):673–8.

[4] Gagner M, Lacroix A, Bolté E. Laparoscopic adrenalectomy in Cushing's syndrome and pheochromocytoma. N Engl J Med. 1992 Oct 1;327(14):1033.

[5] Gagner M, Pomp A, Heniford BT, Pharand D, Lacroix A. Laparoscopic adrenalectomy: lessons learned from 100 consecutive procedures. Ann Surg. 1997 Sep;226(3):238–47.

[6] Bonjer HJ, Sorm V, Berends FJ, Kazemier G, Steyerberg EW, de Herder WW, Bruining HA. Endoscopic retroperitoneal adrenalectomy: lessons learned from 111 consecutive cases. Ann Surg. 2000 Dec;232(6):796–803.

[7] Salomon L, Rabii R, Soulie M, Mouly P, Hoznek A, Cicco A, Saint F, Alame W, Antiphon P, Chopin D, Plante P, Abbou CC. Experience with retroperitoneal laparoscopic adrenalectomy for pheochromocytoma. J Urol. 2001 Jun;165(6 Pt 1):1871–4.

[8] Guerrieri M, Baldarelli M, Scarpelli M, Santini S, Lezoche G, Lezoche E. Laparoscopic adrenalectomy in pheochromocytomas. J Endocrinol Invest. 2005 Jun;28(6):523–7.

[9] Lang B, Fu B, OuYang JZ, Wang BJ, Zhang GX, Xu K, Zhang J, Wang C, Shi TP, Zhou HX, Ma X, Zhang X. Retrospective comparison of retroperitoneoscopic versus open adrenalectomy for pheochromocytoma. J Urol. 2008 Jan;179(1):57–60.

[10] Janetschek G, Finkenstedt G, Gasser R, Waibel UG, Peschel R, Bartsch G, Neumann HP. Laparoscopic surgery for pheochromocytoma: adrenalectomy, partial resection, excision of paragangliomas. J Urol. 1998 Aug;160(2):330–4.

[11] Paganini AM, Guerrieri M, Balla A, Quaresima S, Isidori AM, Iafrate F, D'Ambrosio G, Lezoche G, Lezoche E. Management of adrenal incidentaloma by laparoscopic transperitoneal anterior and submesocolic approach. Langenbecks Arch Surg. 2016 Feb;401(1):71–9. doi:10.1007/s00423-015-1367-y

[12] Thompson GB, Young WF Jr. Adrenal incidentaloma. Curr Opin Oncol. 2003 Jan;15 (1):84–90.

[13] Sahdev A, Reznek RH. Imaging evaluation of the non-functioning indeterminate adrenal mass. Trends Endocrinol Metab. 2004 Aug;15(6):271–6.

[14] Szolar DH, Korobkin M, Reittner P, Berghold A, Bauernhofer T, Trummer H, Schoellnast H, Preidler KW, Samonigg H. Adrenocortical carcinomas and adrenal pheochromocytomas:

mass and enhancement loss evaluation at delayed contrast-enhanced CT. Radiology. 2005 Feb;234(2):479–85.

[15] Young WF Jr. Clinical practice. The incidentally discovered adrenal mass. N Engl J Med. 2007 Feb 8;356(6):601–10.

[16] Lockhart ME, Smith JK, Kenney PJ. Imaging of adrenal masses. Eur J Radiol. 2002 Feb;41 (2):95–112.

[17] Slattery JM, Blake MA, Kalra MK, Misdraji J, Sweeney AT, Copeland PM, Mueller PR, Boland GW. Adrenocortical carcinoma: contrast washout characteristics on CT. AJR Am J Roentgenol. 2006 Jul;187(1):W21–4.

[18] Ilias I, Sahdev A, Reznek RH, Grossman AB, Pacak K. The optimal imaging of adrenal tumours: a comparison of different methods. Endocr Relat Cancer. 2007 Sep;14(3):587–99.

[19] Paganini AM, Balla A, Guerrieri M, Lezoche G, Campagnacci R, D'Ambrosio G, Quaresima S, Antonica MV, Lezoche E. Laparoscopic transperitoneal anterior adrenalectomy in pheochromocytoma: experience in 62 patients. Surg Endosc. 2014 Sep;28 (9):2683–9. doi:10.1007/s00464-014-3528-4

[20] Zacharias M, Haese A, Jurczok A, Stolzenburg JU, Fornara P. Transperitoneal laparoscopic adrenalectomy: outline of the preoperative management, surgical approach, and outcome. Eur Urol. 2006 Mar;49(3):448–59.

[21] Hisano M, Vicentini FC, Srougi M. Retroperitoneoscopic adrenalectomy in pheochromocytoma. Clinics (Sao Paulo). 2012;67(Suppl 1):161–7.

[22] Chen H, Sippel RS, O'Dorisio MS, Vinik AI, Lloyd RV, Pacak K. North American Neuroendocrine Tumor Society (NANETS). The North American Neuroendocrine Tumor Society consensus guideline for the diagnosis and management of neuroendocrine tumors: pheochromocytoma, paraganglioma, and medullary thyroid cancer. Pancreas. 2010 Aug;39(6):775–83. doi:10.1097/MPA.0b013e3181ebb4f0

[23] Feliciotti F, Paganini AM, Guerrieri M, Baldarelli M, De Sanctis A, Campagnacci R, Lezoche E. Laparoscopic anterior adrenalectomy for the treatment of adrenal metastases. Surg Laparosc Endosc Percutan Tech. 2003 Oct;13(5):328–33.

[24] Lezoche E, Guerrieri M, Feliciotti F, Paganini AM, Perretta S, Baldarelli M, Bonjer J, Miccoli P. Anterior, lateral, and posterior retroperitoneal approaches in endoscopic adrenalectomy. Surg Endosc. 2002 Jan;16(1):96–9.

[25] Brunt LM, Doherty GM, Norton JA, Soper NJ, Quasebarth MA, Moley JF. Laparoscopic adrenalectomy compared to open adrenalectomy for benign adrenal neoplasms. J Am Coll Surg. 1996 Jul;183(1):1–10.

[26] Scoglio D, Balla A, Pacilè M, Guerrieri M, Lezoche G, D'Ambrosio G, Fabiani B, Ursi P, Paganini AM. Laparoscopic transperitoneal anterior adrenalectomy. Ann Ital Chir. 2013 Jul-Aug;84(4):411–6.

[27] Mohammadi-Fallah MR, Mehdizadeh A, Badalzadeh A, Izadseresht B, Dadkhah N, Barbod A, Babaie M, Hamedanchi S. Comparison of transperitoneal versus retroperitoneal

laparoscopic adrenalectomy in a prospective randomized study. J Laparoendosc Adv Surg Tech A. 2013 Apr;23(4):362–6. doi:10.1089/lap.2012.0301

[28] Chen W, Li F, Chen D, Zhu Y, He C, Du Y, Tan W. Retroperitoneal versus transperitoneal laparoscopic adrenalectomy in adrenal tumor: a meta-analysis. Surg Laparosc Endosc Percutan Tech. 2013 Apr;23(2):121–7. doi:10.1097/SLE.0b013e3182827b57

[29] Matsuda T, Murota T, Kawakita M. Transperitoneal anterior laparoscopic adrenalectomy: the easiest technique. Biomed Pharmacother. 2000 Jun;54(Suppl 1):157s–60s.

[30] Dickson PV, Alex GC, Grubbs EG, Ayala-Ramirez M, Jimenez C, Evans DB, Lee JE, Perrier ND. Posterior retroperitoneoscopic adrenalectomy is a safe and effective alternative to transabdominal laparoscopic adrenalectomy for pheochromocytoma. Surgery. 2011 Sep;150(3):452–8. doi:10.1016/j.surg.2011.07.004

[31] Fernández-Cruz L, Saenz A, Taura P, Benarroch G, Astudillo E, Sabater L. Retroperitoneal approach in laparoscopic adrenalectomy: is it advantageous? Surg Endosc. 1999 Jan;13 (1):86–90.

[32] Nigri G, Rosman AS, Petrucciani N, Fancellu A, Pisano M, Zorcolo L, Ramacciato G, Melis M. Meta-analysis of trials comparing laparoscopic transperitoneal and retroperitoneal adrenalectomy. Surgery. 2013 Jan;153(1):111–9. doi:10.1016/j.surg.2012.05.042

[33] Walz MK, Alesina PF, Wenger FA, Deligiannis A, Szuczik E, Petersenn S, Ommer A, Groeben H, Peitgen K, Janssen OE, Philipp T, Neumann HP, Schmid KW, Mann K. Posterior retroperitoneoscopic adrenalectomy--results of 560 procedures in 520 patients. Surgery. 2006 Dec;140(6):943–50.

[34] Prager G, Heinz-Peer G, Passler C, Kaczirek K, Schindl M, Scheuba C, Niederle B. Surgical strategy in adrenal masses. Eur J Radiol. 2002 Jan;41(1):70–7.

[35] Benedetti-Valentini S, Rossodivita I. Delbet's submesocolic approach for surgery of the left adrenal gland. Osp Ital Chir. 1968 Mar;18(3):285–8.

[36] Janetschek G, Neumann HP. Laparoscopic surgery for pheochromocytoma. Urol Clin North Am. 2001 Feb;28(1):97–105.

[37] Lezoche E, Guerrieri M, Crosta F, Lezoche G, Baldarelli M, Campagnacci R. Flank approach versus anterior sub-mesocolic access in left laparoscopic adrenalectomy: a prospective randomized study. Surg Endosc. 2008 Nov;22(11):2373–8. doi:10.1007/s00464-008-9783-5

[38] Col V, de Cannière L, Collard E, Michel L, Donckier J. Laparoscopic adrenalectomy for phaeochromocytoma: endocrinological and surgical aspects of a new therapeutic approach. Clin Endocrinol (Oxf). 1999 Jan;50(1):121–5.

[39] Flávio Rocha M, Faramarzi-Roques R, Tauzin-Fin P, Vallee V, Leitao de Vasconcelos PR, Ballanger P. Laparoscopic surgery for pheochromocytoma. Eur Urol. 2004 Feb;45 (2):226–32.

[40] Cobb WS, Kercher KW, Sing RF, Heniford BT. Laparoscopic adrenalectomy for malignancy. Am J Surg. 2005 Apr;189(4):405–11.

[41] Godellas CV, Prinz RA. Surgical approach to adrenal neoplasms: laparoscopic versus open adrenalectomy. Surg Oncol Clin N Am. 1998 Oct;7(4):807–17.

[42] Parnaby CN, Chong PS, Chisholm L, Farrow J, Connell JM, O'Dwyer PJ. The role of laparoscopic adrenalectomy for adrenal tumours of 6 cm or greater. Surg Endosc. 2008 Mar;22(3):617–21.

[43] Lucas SW, Spitz JD, Arregui ME. The use of intraoperative ultrasound in laparoscopic adrenal surgery: the Saint Vincent experience. Surg Endosc. 1999 Nov;13(11):1093–8.

[44] Cabalag MS, Mann GB, Gorelik A, Miller JA. Comparison of outcomes after laparoscopic versus posterior retroperitoneoscopic adrenalectomy: a pilot study. Surg Laparosc Endosc Percutan Tech. 2014 Feb;24(1):62–6. doi:10.1097/SLE.0b013e31828fa71f

[45] Linos DA, Stylopoulos N, Boukis M, Souvatzoglou A, Raptis S, Papadimitriou J. Anterior, posterior, or laparoscopic approach for the management of adrenal diseases? Am J Surg. 1997 Feb;173(2):120–5.

[46] Sound S, Okoh AK, Bucak E, Yigitbas H, Dural C, Berber E. Intraoperative tumor localization and tissue distinction during robotic adrenalectomy using indocyanine green fluorescence imaging: a feasibility study. Surg Endosc. 2016 Feb;30(2):657–62. doi:10.1007/s00464-015-4256-0

[47] DeLong JC, Chakedis JM, Hosseini A, Kelly KJ, Horgan S, Bouvet M. Indocyanine green (ICG) fluorescence-guided laparoscopic adrenalectomy. J Surg Oncol. 2015 Nov;112 (6):650–3. doi:10.1002/jso.24057

[48] Constantinides VA, Christakis I, Touska P, Palazzo FF. Systematic review and meta-analysis of retroperitoneoscopic versus laparoscopic adrenalectomy. Br J Surg. 2012 Dec;99(12):1639–48. doi:10.1002/bjs.8921

Chapter 5

Ergonomics in Laparoscopic Surgery

Francisco M. Sánchez-Margallo and

Juan A. Sánchez-Margallo

Additional information is available at the end of the chapter

http://dx.doi.org/10.5772/66170

Abstract

Despite the many advantages for patients, laparoscopic surgery entails certain ergonomic inconveniences for surgeons, which may result in decreasing the surgeons' performance and musculoskeletal disorders. In this chapter, the current status of ergonomics in laparoscopy, laparoendoscopic single-site surgery (LESS), and robot-assisted surgery will be reviewed. Ergonomic guidelines for laparoscopic surgical practice and methods for ergonomic assessment in surgery will be described. Results will be based on the scientific literature and our experience. Results showed that the surgeon's posture during laparoscopic surgery is mainly affected by the static body postures, the height of the operating table, the design of the surgical instruments, the position of the main screen, and the use of foot pedals. Ergonomics during the laparoscopic surgical practice is related to the level of experience. Better ergonomic conditions entail an improvement in task performance. Laparoscopic instruments with axial handle lead to a more ergonomic posture for the wrist compared to a ring handle. LESS is physically more demanding than conventional and hybrid approaches, requiring greater level of muscular activity in the back and arm muscles, but better wrist position compared with traditional laparoscopy. Physical and cognitive ergonomics with robotic assistance were significantly less challenging when compared to conventional laparoscopic surgery.

Keywords: Ergonomics, laparoscopic surgery, laparoendoscopic single-site surgery, robotic instrument, electromyography, motion capture

1. Introduction

Despite the many advantages for patients, laparoscopic surgery entails certain ergonomic inconveniences for surgeons, namely, loss of freedom during surgical maneuvers, deriving in an increased incidence of static postures, and adoption and maintenance of forced body postures for long periods of time. Since laparoscopic surgery became more advanced, operating time expanded and, in proportion, so did the levels of mental and physical stress imposed on the surgical team [1]. The combination of these factors with inadequate ergonomic design of surgical instruments may result in decreasing the surgeons' performance and accuracy, as well as the incidence of physical fatigue and musculoskeletal disorders.

The main technical limitations of laparoscopic surgery come from the technical modifications with regard to the open approach. Visual displays are located apart from the surgical field, affecting hand-eye coordination. Furthermore, bidimensional vision causes a confusing loss of depth perception. Specific instruments and fixed access ports limit movements and tactile feedback, worsening surgical performance and demanding greater muscular activity [2]. Design of laparoscopic tools implies a high degree of complexity, requiring manual skills and complementary new knowledge of how to use them. Design of surgical instruments and medical devices, as well as specific location of the monitor, operating table, foot pedals, and other surgical equipment determine to a large extent surgeons' postures while performing surgical procedures and the organization of the surgical team.

The introduction of laparoendoscopic single-site surgery (LESS) has led to a reduction of the number and size of incisions, thus providing aesthetical and emotional improvements to the patients. Positive results have been reported for this surgical approach with regard to postoperative outcomes, recovery time, length of hospital stay, and related costs [3]. LESS inherits the constraints of conventional laparoscopic surgery, adding new technical challenges. Working through a single port implies a defective triangulation, even more lack of coordination, external and internal instrument clashing, forced hands approximation with restrained manipulation, narrowing of the operative field, and possible pneumoperitoneum leakage [4]. Therefore, the use of LESS approach leads to a greater physical and mental workload for the surgeons [5, 6].

Robotic surgery is an increasingly expanding technology that uses human-machine interfaces providing solutions to laparoscopic constraints through enhanced dexterity, maneuverability, stability, and accuracy. Several studies reported lower complication rates and blood loss than conventional laparoscopic surgery [7]. This technology has been also integrated with LESS, and even more complex procedures by means of flexible access devices [8]. The main limitations of robotic surgery are high expenses and maintenance costs, difficulty to use it in low-volume or low-income centers, required experience from the surgical team, and instruments replacement [9].

The term ergonomics can be defined as the scientific study of humans at labor. The main objective of this field is to adapt environments to workers, improving equipment, workplaces, productivity, and training [10]. In this respect, ergonomics applied to laparoscopic surgery is focused on instruments' design and ergonomic assessment, surgeons' posture and workload

analysis, surgical environment, and visual displays development [11, 12]. The main objective of this chapter is to review and analyze the ergonomic conditions during laparoscopic surgery and novel minimally invasive surgical approaches such as LESS and robotic surgery, as well as to establish ergonomic guidelines for laparoscopic surgical practice. In order to reach more representative information, studies published after 2010 and with over 20 subjects will be taken into account, excluding the review articles. The content of this chapter will be organized in three main sections: general ergonomic aspects in laparoscopic surgery, methods and technologies for ergonomic assessment in surgery, and ergonomics in minimally invasive surgical approaches.

2. General aspects

In laparoscopic surgery there are some primary ergonomic risk factors for the surgeon such as the body posture, the organization of the work space in the operating room (OR), and the design of the surgical tools.

2.1. Body posture

Laparoscopic surgery has changed the way surgeons interact in the operating field, what is revealed by a change in their posture and movements mainly of the upper limbs. In laparoscopic surgery dexterity is limited due to the fixed access port position, determining the angle of the instruments and instruments motion. Degrees of freedom are restricted from 36 in open surgery to 4 in laparoscopic surgery. This limited range of action leads to surgeons to acquire static, forced, and awkward long-term postures. The primary risk factor for the appearing of musculoskeletal disorders is body deviation from the neutral position. The ideal position for the laparoscopic surgeon is characterized by the arms slightly abducted, retroverted, and rotated inward at the shoulder level; the elbow should be bent at a 90–120° angle; the hands should grasp the instruments with the wrist slightly extended and with the distal interphalangeal joints almost extended, and the metacarpophalangeal and proximal interphalangeal joints flexed at 30–50°; fingers should be abducted and the thumb should be opposed to the index finger [13, 14]. Surgical team and equipment location in relation to the patient also must be considered. Likewise, lower body position can be non-ergonomic, provoking physical stress. Surgeons usually perform long procedures standing with a potential loss of stability and limited possibilities to change their body weight, especially when foot pedals are used [15].

2.2. Working environment

The workplace organization means that every individual member of the surgical team has appropriate space and access to all equipment. A lack of balance between the surgical staff and OR components can lead to work overloads and injuries. The advances in the field of laparoscopy are reflected in the development of optics with higher resolution and improved operational instruments. However, this progress has not always been accompanied by an ergonomic upgrade, which would alleviate some of the problems experienced by laparoscopic

surgeons. Besides, some considerations have to be taken into account when using the laparoscopic equipment before and during surgical procedures.

2.2.1. *The monitor*

The visual information from the surgical scenario is provided by a monitor, which should be adjusted prior to the surgery to avoid undesirable postures for a long period of time. In the horizontal plane, the monitor should be straight ahead of the surgeon and in line with the forearm–instrument motor axis. In the sagittal plain, it should be positioned lower than the surgeon's eye level to avoid neck extension. The most comfortable viewing direction is approximately 15° downward. Viewing distance is highly dependent on monitor size. It should be far enough to avoid extensive accommodation of the eyes and contraction by the extraocular muscles, and close enough to avoid staring and loss of detail [16, 17]. To accomplish precision tasks, the use of an additional monitor near the operative field is recommended, as it improves hand-eye coordination [12, 17].

2.2.2. *Operating table*

The operating table must be adapted to the surgeon's height and position (standing or sitting). If the operating table is placed too high, muscles apply considerably more contraction force in order to raise and hold the shoulders as well as the elbows. If that position is maintained for a period of time it leads quickly to shoulder muscles fatigue. The table's height should be adjusted in such a way that laparoscopic instrument handles are slightly below the level of the surgeon's elbows. The proper table location keeps shoulders down, and the angle between the lower and upper arm is between 90° and 120° when performing manual work [18, 19]. Lifts can be used in case the table cannot be lowered to a certain height.

2.2.3. *Foot pedals*

Foot pedals are commonly used during laparoscopic surgery to activate instruments such as electrocauterization, ultrasonic shears, bipolar device, or other tissue welding/dividing instruments. They are often poorly positioned and could demand awkward and unnatural postures. Their main problems are the lack of visual control, unbalanced position of the surgeon, and use of too many pedals during laparoscopic surgery. A possible solution could be replacing them with hand controls when possible. Pedals should be placed near the foot and aligned in the same direction as the instruments, toward the target quadrant and laparoscopic monitor. This allows surgeons to activate the pedal without twisting their body or leg. A pedal with a built-in foot rest is preferable [20].

2.2.4. *Surgical instruments*

The performance of laparoscopic procedures and the position of surgeon's arms, hands, and fingers are highly dependent on the design of surgical instruments, mainly on the shape of the handle and the tool length. The non-ergonomic designs of handles that are not adapted to the shape and size of the surgeon's hand may lead to discomfort, paresthesias of the digital nerves

and muscle fatigue [13]. Surgical instruments should enable surgeons to minimize the wrist flexion and rotation and ulnar deviation, keeping both arms at the sides of their body, and avoiding pressure points on their hands and fingers. Design of instrument handle should be according to the task to be performed, pistol-type handle for tasks that required force and precision-type handle for tasks that require precision [20].

3. Methods for ergonomic assessment

3.1. Body posture

The analysis of the interaction between the surgeon and surgical environment is a determinant factor to evaluate the ergonomic suitability of the working environment and provides crucial information to establish its basic design features. Traditional methods to assess surgeon's postures associated with a specific surgical activity have been based on observation techniques (photogrammetry) by observing the subject directly or using a recorded video [21, 22]. However, assessment methods have evolved and currently it is possible to perform and ergonomic analysis in the OR and using more automated technology. In this section, different methods of ergonomic assessment will be described based on kinematic analysis, muscle activity, or mental stress.

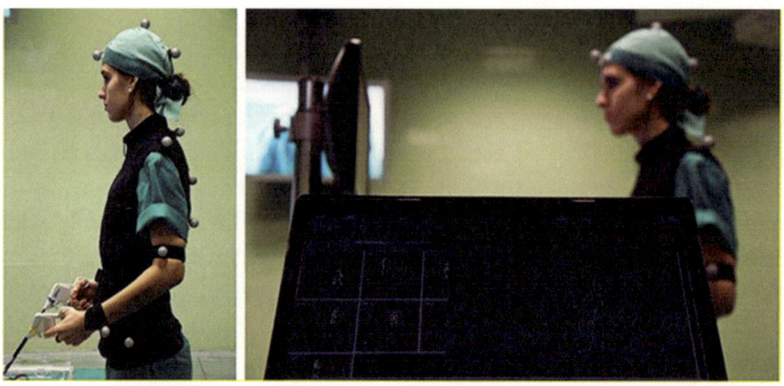

Figure 1. Motion tracking system based on retro-reflective markers. Artificial markers are placed on the targeted segments of the surgeon's body (*left*). A software application computes the kinematics variables during the task execution (*right*).

3.1.1. 3D motion tracking

These measurement systems quantify human movements by means of positional data obtained from artificial markers or sensors placed on the subject's body. Optical tracking techniques are based on color or retro-reflective markers that are identified at the three-dimensional space by a set of cameras [23] around the working space (**Figure 1**). However, these markers may have some occlusion problems in crowded spaces such as the OR, mainly because of the surgical

staff and equipment. Another technology for motion tracking is the use of inertial sensors to record in real time the different body segments for subsequent kinematic analysis (**Figure 2**). These inertial measurement units are not affected by visual occlusions, and thus are appropriate for working environments as the OR.

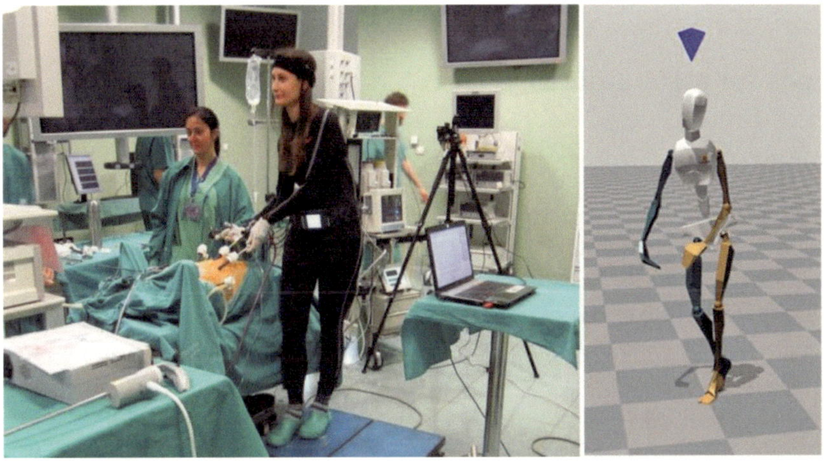

Figure 2. Motion tracking system based on inertial sensors embedded in an elastic suit (*left*). A biomechanical model of the subject is created in real time (*right*).

A set of kinematics variables such as translational and rotational positions, velocities, and accelerations can be computed using the recorded positional data of the subject. Afterwards, the surgeon's posture can be analyzed with standard evaluation techniques such as Rapid Upper Limb Assessment (RULA) method or Ovako Working Analysis System (OWAS). Youssef et al. [24] compared variations in the surgeon's standing position during a virtual reality-simulated laparoscopic cholecystectomy using RULA score. They obtained better ergonomic posture for the between-standing technique, regardless of whether one- or two-handed technique. 3D kinematic analysis was used to differentiate joint variability between conventional laparoscopy and LESS [21], evaluating the influence of the upper body to the head stabilization.

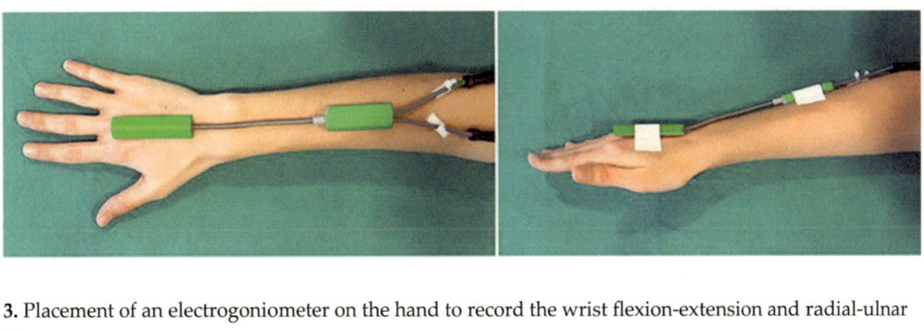

Figure 3. Placement of an electrogoniometer on the hand to record the wrist flexion-extension and radial-ulnar deviation.

http://dx.doi.org/10.5772/66170

3.1.2. Electrogoniometers

Electrogoniometers are devices whose measurement signals (typically electrical voltages) are related directly to flexion-extension or rotation between body segments. These devices should be precalibrated to relate the measured voltage with the angles described by the analyzed joint (**Figure 3**). However, this measurement technology may be difficult to use for certain body segments. Besides, the need to be attached to the body segments and the use of wires for power supply make these devices a cumbersome solution to be used during laparoscopic practice.

3.1.3. Data gloves

Surgical tasks and instruments directly affect the surgeon's wrist and hand position. Data gloves allow for recording movements of the fingers and wrist by means of electromechanical technology or conductive sensors. In the clinical field, these devices have been used in conjunction with virtual reality systems for rehabilitation purposes [25] and surgical planning applications [26]. Recently, this technology has been used to analyze the surgeon's hand movements while using different surgical instruments during laparoscopic practice [5, 8, 11, 27] (**Figure 4**).

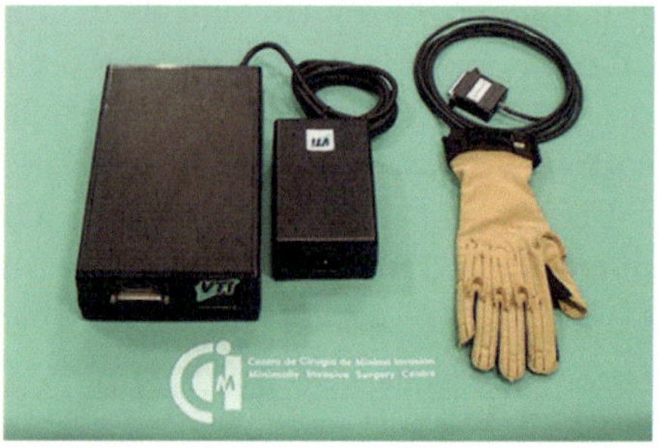

Figure 4. Motion capture data glove CyberGlove® (CyberGlove Systems, San José, CA, USA). This device consists of a series of conductive sensors with resistance flows sensitive to flexion variations.

3.2. Electromyography

Electromyography (EMG) measures the electrical signal associated with the activation of the muscle. This technique allows us to assess the electrical activity of a muscle group during the performance of a task. For data acquisition, electrodes should be placed following standard recommendations, as the surface EMG for noninvasive assessment of muscles (SENIAM) project [28], to ensure the acquisition of EMG signals and reduce potential artifacts.

Several metrics of muscle activity during the execution of a certain task can be computed by analyzing the EMG signal such as the percentage of the maximal voluntary contraction (MVC) [29], the amplitude probability distribution function (APDF) [30], or the muscle fatigue [6]. EMG has been an extended ergonomic assessment method in laparoscopic surgery to analyze

the surgeon's postural muscle activity [5, 11], the use of different surgical instruments, and instrument handles [27, 31] (**Figure 5**).

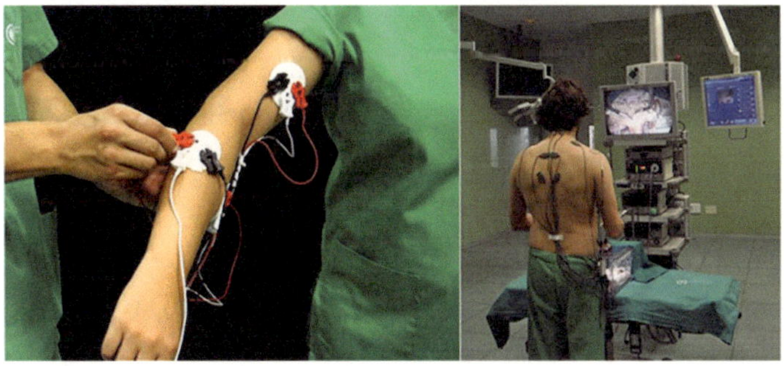

Figure 5. Placement of the EMG electrodes on the right biceps brachii and forearm extensors (*left*). Use of the surface EMG to analyze the muscle activity of the upper body during laparoscopic practice (*right*).

3.3. Force platforms

Force platforms (single or multiple) are used to analyze the body balance during static or dynamic situations. These systems provide information about ground's reaction force against the force exerted by the subject's legs while supporting the body weight. Fan et al. [32] presented an alternative position to conventional flank position in retroperitoneoscopic urological practice. Body balance was assessed during simulated surgical tasks using two separate force plates (Wii Fit balance boards, Nintendo Inc.). They concluded that relative loading between feet was more balanced using the purposed posture.

3.4. Mental workload

Apart from the physical effort, psychological burden of surgeons performing laparoscopic procedures is reported higher in comparison to open surgical techniques [15]. For mental workload assessment, subjective techniques are the most extended methods. The National Aeronautics and Space Administration Task Load Index (NASA-TLX) evaluates six domains: mental demand, physical demand, temporal demand, effort, performance, and frustration during each task execution. A surgery-specific version of the NASA-TLX called SURG-TLX was presented and validated in 2011 [33]. Apart from the physical, mental, and temporal demand, this index assessed the task complexity, the situational stress, and distractions. Studies reported LESS is significantly more demanding than the conventional approach [34]. Training has been proved to improve both task performance and workload in laparoscopic practice [35].

3.5. Questionnaires

Questionnaires are another assessment tool that focuses on gathering information from a population of surgeons. Taking into account studies with at least 100 respondents, a survey

to laparoscopic urologists in China concluded that most of them were not aware of the ergonomic guidelines for the OR [36]. Shoulder, neck, back, and hand pain and stiffness were reported as the main physical symptoms during laparoscopic procedures [36, 37]. The surgeon's height, glove size, age, gender, type of instrument, foot pedals, and height of the operating table have been identified as important factors for increasing the musculoskeletal pain symptoms [38–41]. The shape of the laparoscopic instrument handle was identified as the main element that needed to be improved [40].

4. Ergonomics in laparoscopic surgery

A summary of the results from the scientific literature regarding ergonomics in laparoscopic surgery are presented in **Table 1**.

Study	*N*	Task	Assessment method	Results
[12]	24 novices	Peg transfer with different monitor conditions	NASA-TLX	There are no differences among monitor positions in terms of perceived workload
[16]	20 novices	Suturing on simulator with ergonomic (G1) and normal (G2) settings	Photogrammetry: Neck, shoulder, elbow, and wrist	Optimal ergonomic setting leads to better task performance
[24]	32	Cholecystectomy on virtual simulator with variations in standing position and hand technique	RULA NASA-TLX	Better ergonomic posture for the between-standing technique [30]
[30]	25	Open, laparoscopic, and endovascular procedures	EMG: Back, neck, and shoulder	Open surgery imposes greater physical demand on the neck muscles compared with endovascular and laparoscopic surgeries
[42]	26: 13 with training of the non-dominant upper extremity and 13 without training	Eye-hand coordination task	EMG: Back, shoulder, and forearm	Training the non-dominant upper extremity leads to better alternated use of forearm muscles
[43]	100	Laparoscopic renal procedures with and without foot gel pad	Subjective criteria	The use of foot gel pads improves surgeon comfort and ergonomics during laparoscopy
[44]	28 novices	Nissen fundoplication model	NASA-TLX	Higher mental workload is associated with poorer laparoscopic performance

N: Number of subjects or cases.

Table 1. Reported results for ergonomics in laparoscopic surgery.

In a study with 30 surgeons with different experience in laparoscopic surgery, we analyzed the surgeon's muscle activity in back and forearm muscles during laparoscopic dissection and suturing tasks [29]. Percentage of the MVC of the trapezius, forearm flexors, and forearm extensors muscles was used for assessment of the muscle activity (**Figure 6**). Results showed that the surgeons with a higher degree of laparoscopic experience exhibited a lower level of muscle activity when compared with the novice surgeons. In another study with 50 surgeons, we analyzed the surgeons' hand spatial configuration during the use of two laparoscopic instrument handles, axial and ring-handled [11]. Movements of the surgeon's hand and wrist were recorded by a data glove and the level of wrist disorder was computed by a modified version of the RULA method [27] (**Figure 6**). Results showed that axial-handled needle holder entailed a more ergonomic posture for the wrist joint.

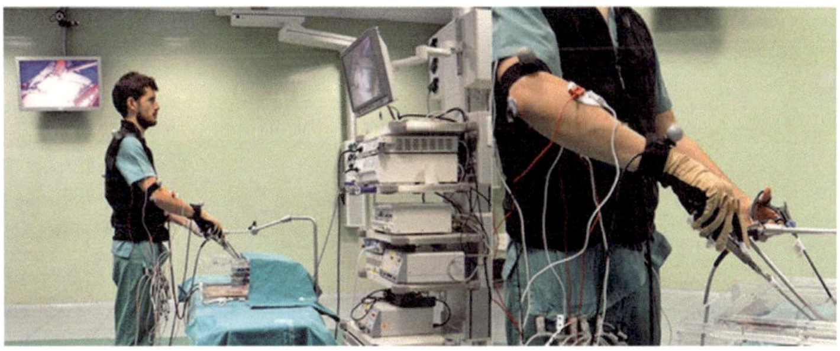

Figure 6. EMG and data glove data acquisition during the performance of laparoscopic tasks on simulator.

5. New surgical approaches

New surgical approaches have been presented to improve surgical outcomes and aesthetics results of patients. However, in some cases these surgical alternatives lead to an increase in technical and ergonomic challenges for surgeons that should be analyzed and identified.

5.1. Laparoendoscopic single-site surgery (LESS)

A summary of the results from the scientific literature for ergonomics in LESS are presented in **Table 2**.

In a study with experienced laparoscopic surgeons we assessed the surgeons' ergonomy during LESS, comparing it with conventional laparoscopic approach [5]. Surgeons performed a dissection tasks on a physical simulator using straight laparoscopic scissors and dissector for the conventional approach, and articulating tip scissors and dissector for the LESS approach (**Figure 7**). Ergonomic assessment was carried out by analyzing the muscular activity, and wrist and hand motion. Results showed that the LESS approach required greater level of muscular activity in the trapezius and forearm extensor muscles, but better wrist position compared with traditional laparoscopy.

Study	*N*	Task	Assessment method	Results
[34]	48: 25 with LESS and 23 with conventional approach	Cholecystectomy	SURG-TLX	LESS cholecystectomy is more stressful and physically demanding than the conventional approach
[45]	24 premedical college students	Peg-transfer with two articulated and one straight graspers	EMG: Forearms. Electrogoniometers: Wrist. SURG-TLX	The straight instrument requires less muscle activation and wrist deviation
[46]	100 procedures: 50 triportal vs. 50 uniportal	Video-assisted thoracic surgery	Photogrammetry: Head NASA-TLX	Surgeons maintain a more neutral body posture during uniportal VATS, but with greater frustration
[47]	90 patients	Laparoscopic pull-through Soave procedure: conventional, LESS and hybrid approach	Subjective criteria	The conventional and hybrid approach have the same maneuverability and are less challenging than the LESS approach
[48]	175 patients	Different urological procedures	Subjective criteria	The use of conventional laparoscopic instruments is ergonomically feasible and safe in LESS procedures

N: Number of subjects or cases.

Table 2. Reported results for ergonomics in LESS.

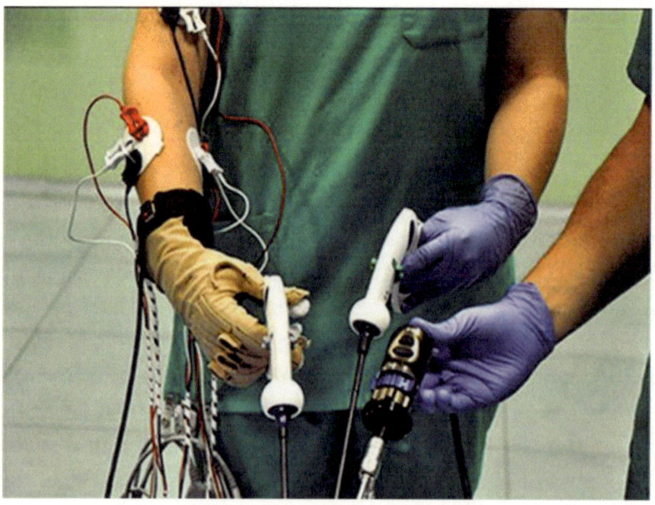

Figure 7. EMG and data glove data acquisition during the performance of hands-on simulator tasks using a LESS approach.

5.2. Robotic surgery

Research has demonstrated the benefits of robotic surgery for the patient such as smaller incisions, reduced blood loss and postoperative pain, and reduced durations of in-patient care. Robotic platforms such as the da Vinci system (Intuitive Surgical Ltd., Sunnyvale, CA, USA) have been presented as a potential solution to the limited ergonomics in laparoscopic surgery.

In a study with surgeons with different levels of experience in robotic surgery, physical and cognitive ergonomic workloads using robotic-assisted and conventional laparoscopy were assessed during the performance of different basic laparoscopic training tasks [49]. Physical workload was assessed by using EMG from back, shoulder, arms, and forearms muscles, and mental workload by means of NASA-TLX index. They concluded that physical and cognitive ergonomics with robotic assistance were significantly less challenging. Another study comparing the use of standard laparoscopy and robotic assistance during intracorporeal suturing on porcine Nissen fundoplication models, medical students reported a lower workload using the robotic assistance [50]. Similarly, Moore et al. [51] reported significantly lower workload and mental effort on the robotic system compared to conventional laparoscopic approach while performing an eye-hand coordination task. Besides, another study using standard laparoscopic tasks during five consecutive training sessions, surgeons (novices and experienced) reported a less frustration score during and after training sessions and higher good mood score using robotic assistance [52]. The Imperial Test Assessment Tool was use to evaluate the frustration level.

6. New surgical devices

In order to overcome some of the ergonomic limitations of laparoscopic surgery, new surgical devices and instrument designs have been developed. In this section, we will review these novel surgical devices presented in the scientific literature. Studies published after 2010 and with no limit of subjects will be taken into account, excluding the review articles.

Several authors presented novel prototypes of ergonomically designed handles for laparoscopic instruments. One example is the Intuitool® laparoscopic instrument (University of Nebraska, Lincoln, NE, USA), which includes an ergonomic handle and a redesigned grasper actuation mechanism in order to create a more comfortable and intuitive handle-tool interface [53]. Büchel et al. [31] also presented a laparoscopic instrument prototype with an ergonomic pistol handle (Volargrip; University Hospital of Trondheim and Surgitech Norway AS, Trondheim, Norway). They compared this tool with two conventional laparoscopic instruments with ring handles. Results showed that each handle except the new prototype caused pressure areas and pain. A pistol grip laparoscopic instrument with a rotatable handle piece was presented by Steinhilber et al. [54]. EMG of the arm and shoulder muscles and wrist's posture by means of a gravimetric posture sensor were used to compare this novel instrument with the use of a conventional laparoscopic handle during the performance of a hand-eye coordination task. Results showed that the novel handle design did not decrease the biomechanical stress of the analyzed muscles, but neutral position of the wrist was more

often. Yu et al. [55] compared a prototype laparoscopic grasper with three adjustable handle angles to a conventional instrument during the performance of Fundamentals of Laparoscopic Surgery tasks. Motion tracking and NASA-TLX were used to measure the surgeon's posture and workload. They concluded that the adjustable handle angle laparoscopic tool can reduce ergonomic risks of musculoskeletal strain and allows versatility for tasks alternating between positions.

Another possibility to improve the ergonomics in laparoscopy is by increasing the instrument's degrees of freedom. This is the case of the Radius Surgical System (Tuebingen Scientific Medical GmbH, Tuebingen, Germany), which provides two additional degrees of freedom (deflection and rotation of the tip) and enables the surgeon to manipulate the instrument accurately and precisely in an ergonomic position [56]. This manipulator has been successfully used to treat cases of esophageal achalasia and gastroesophageal reflux disease [57].

Apart from laparoscopic surgical instruments, other support devices have been developed to improve the ergonomic conditions during surgery. This is the case of operating chairs [58] or arm supports [59], whose main objective is to improve the surgeon's ergonomic posture during surgery. A novel portable ergonomic simulator for training of basic laparoscopic skills was also presented by Xiao et al. [60].

6.1. Handheld robotic instruments

New handheld robotic systems have been developed for laparoscopic surgery and single-site surgery to deal with some of their technical and ergonomic limitations. They provide precision-driven and articulating instrument tips, which increase the triangulation, and therefore improve the performance of some surgical maneuvers. One example of these systems is Jaimy® (Endocontrol, Grenoble, France), which provides two additional degrees of freedom controlled by a joystick placed on an ergonomic handle [8]. This handheld robotic instrument was ergonomically compared by means of surgeon's posture and muscular activity analysis with a conventional needle holder during the performance of basic laparoscopic training tasks. Results showed that the use of the robotized needle holder improved the surgeon's posture when compared to the traditional laparoscopic instrument.

The Kymerax™ (Terumo Europe NV, Leuven, Belgium) and DEX™ (Dextérité Surgical, Annecy, France) are other examples of handled robotic instruments for laparoscopic surgery and LESS. We have analyzed the ergonomics of these two surgical devices and compared it to conventional laparoscopic instruments by means of motion tracking, EMG of back, shoulder, and arm muscles, and data glove motion analysis (**Figure 8**). A positive learning curve in performance and ergonomics using the handheld robotic instruments has been reported. There were no differences in surgeon's muscle activity using the robotic and the conventional laparoscopic instruments, except for the biceps muscle. The robotic instruments led to an ergonomically more acceptable posture of the shoulder, elbow, and wrist. We believe that a period of adaptation should be required for this new technology.

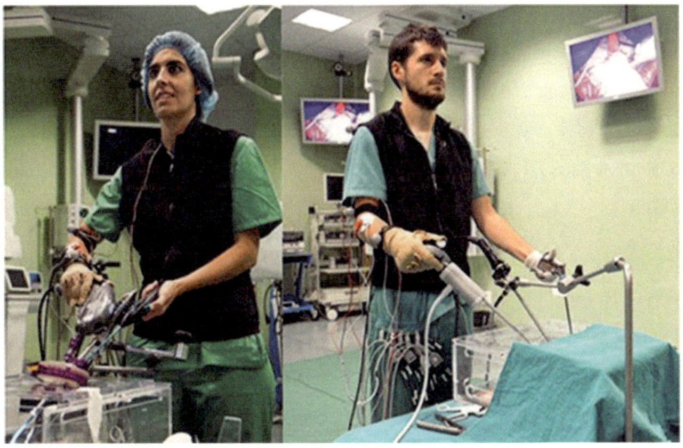

Figure 8. Setup for the ergonomic study in the training environment using (left) the Kymerax™ and (right) the DEX™ handheld robotic instruments.

7. Conclusions

Laparoscopic surgery entails a limited range of movements, which leads to acquire static, forced, and awkward long-term postures. The primary risk factor for the appearing of musculoskeletal disorders is body deviation from the neutral position. The ideal position for the laparoscopic surgeon is characterized by the arms slightly abducted, retroverted, and rotated inward at the shoulder level; the elbow should be bent at a 90–120° angle; the hands should grasp the instruments with the wrist slightly extended. Results from the scientific literature showed that ergonomics during the laparoscopic surgical practice is related to the level of experience. Better ergonomic conditions during surgery lead to an improvement in task performance. Objective ergonomic analysis concluded that laparoscopic instruments with axial handel entail a more ergonomic posture for the wrist joint compared to a ring handle. Regarding ergonomics in LESS, studies reported that this surgical approach is more physically demanding than conventional and hybrid approaches. LESS approach requires greater level of muscular activity in the back and arm muscles, but leads to a better wrist position compared with traditional laparoscopy. Physical and cognitive ergonomics with robotic assistance were significantly less challenging when compared to conventional laparoscopic surgery. Further studies with a greater number of subjects should be done in order to obtain clear evidence-based findings of ergonomics during minimally invasive surgery.

Acknowledgements

This study was supported by the Government of Extremadura, Spain; the European Regional Development Fund (GR15175); and the European Social Fund (PO14034).

Author details

Francisco M. Sánchez-Margallo[1] and Juan A. Sánchez-Margallo[2*]

*Address all correspondence to: juan.sanchez.margallo@gmail.com

1 Jesús Usón Minimally Invasive Surgery Centre, Cáceres, Spain

2 Department of Computer Systems and Telematics Engineering, University of Extremadura, Badajoz, Spain

References

[1] Vereczkel A, Bupp H, Feussner H. Laparoscopic surgery and ergonomics—it's time to think on ourselves as well. Surg Endosc 2003; 17: 1680–2.

[2] Pérez-Duarte FJ, Sánchez-Margallo FM, Díaz-Güemes I, Sánchez-Hurtado MÁ, Lucas-Hernández M, Usón J. Ergonomics in laparoscopic surgery and its importance in surgical training. Cir Esp 2012; 90: 284–91.

[3] Geng L, Sun C, Bai J. Single incision versus conventional laparoscopic cholecystectomy outcomes: a meta-analysis of randomized controlled trials. PLoS One 2013; 8(10): e76530.

[4] Matos-Azevedo AM, Díaz-Guëmes I, Pérez-Duarte FJ, Sánchez-Hurtado MÁ, Sánchez-Margallo FM. Comparison of single access devices during cut and suturing tasks on simulator. J Surg Res 2014; 192(2): 356–67.

[5] Pérez-Duarte FJ, Lucas-Hernández M, Matos-Azevedo A, Sánchez-Margallo JA, Díaz-Güemes I, Sánchez-Margallo FM. Objective analysis of surgeons' ergonomy during laparoendoscopic single-site surgery through the use of surface electromyography and a motion capture data glove. Surg Endosc 2014; 28: 1314–20.

[6] Koca D, Yıldız S, Soyupek F, Günyeli İ, Erdemoglu E, Soyupek S, et al. Physical and mental workload in single-incision laparoscopic surgery and conventional laparoscopy. Surg Innov 2015; 22(3): 294–302.

[7] Ficarra V, Novara G, Artibani W, Cestari A, Galfano A, Graefen M, et al. Retropubic, laparoscopic, and robot-assisted radical prostatectomy: a systematic review and cumulative analysis of comparative studies. Eur Urol 2009; 55: 1037–63.

[8] Bensignor T, Morel G, Reversat D, Fuks D, Gayet B. Evaluation of the effect of a laparoscopic robotized needle holder on ergonomics and skills. Surg Endosc 2016; 30: 446–54.

[9] Elhage O, Challacombe B, Shortland A, Dasgupta P. An assessment of the physical impact of complex surgical tasks on surgeon errors and discomfort: a comparison

between robot-assisted, laparoscopic and open approaches. BJU Int 2015; 115(2): 274–81.

[10] Supe AN, Kulkarni GV, Supe PA. Ergonomics in laparoscopic surgery. J Min Access Surg 2010; 6: 31–6.

[11] Sánchez-Margallo FM, Pérez-Duarte FJ, Sánchez-Margallo JA, Lucas-Hernández M, Matos-Azevedo AM, Díaz-Güemes I. Application of a motion capture data glove for hand and wrist ergonomic analysis during laparoscopy. Minim Invasive Ther Allied Technol 2014; 23(6): 350–6.

[12] Rogers ML, Heath WB, Uy CC, Suresh S, Kaber DB. Effect of visual displays and locations on laparoscopic surgical training task. Appl Ergon 2012; 43: 762–7.

[13] Matern U, Waller P. Instruments for minimally invasive surgery. Principles of ergonomic handles. Surg Endosc 2009; 13: 174–82.

[14] Matern U. Ergonomic deficiencies in the operating room: examples from minimally invasive surgery. Work 2009; 32: 1–4.

[15] Gofrit ON, Mikahail AA, Zorn KC, Zagaja GP, Steinberg GD, Shalhav AL. Surgeons' perceptions and injuries during and after urologic laparoscopic surgery. Urology 2008; 71: 404–7.

[16] Xiao DJ, Jakimowicz JJ, Albayrak A, Goossens RHM. Ergonomic factors on task performance in laparoscopic surgery training. Appl Ergonom 2012; 43: 548–53.

[17] Van Det MJ, Meijerink WJHJ, Hoff C, Totté ER, Pierie JPEN. Optimal ergonomics for laparoscopic surgery in minimally invasive surgery suites: a review and guidelines. Surg Endosc 2009; 23: 1279–85.

[18] Berquer R, Smith WD, Davis S. An ergonomic study of the optimum operating table height for laparoscopic surgery. Surg Endosc 2002;16: 416–21.

[19] Van Veelen MA, Kazemier G, Koopman J, Goossens RH, Meijer DW. Assessment of the ergonomically optimal operating surface height for laparoscopic surgery. J Laparoendosc Adv Surg Technol A 2002; 12(1): 47–52.

[20] Berguer R. Ergonomics in laparoscopic surgery. In: Whelan RL, Fleshman JW, Fowler DL, editors. The SAGES Manual of Perioperative Care in Minimally Invasive Surgery. 2005. New York: Springer. pp. 454–64.

[21] Gianikellis K, Sánchez-Margallo FM, Skiadopoulos A, Sánchez-Margallo JA, Aranda JH de M. Head stabilization during minimal invasive surgery tasks: an uncontrolled manifold analysis. Procedia Manuf 2015; 3: 1434–41.

[22] Gianikellis K, Skiadopoulos A, Palma CE, Sanchez-Margallo FM, Carrasco JBP, Sanchez-Margallo JA. A method to assess upper-body postural variability in laparoscopic surgery. 5th IEEE RAS/EMBS International Conference on Biomedical Robotics and Biomechatronics, IEEE; 2014, pp. 76–81.

[23] Lee G, Lee T, Dexter D, Klein R, Park A. Methodological infrastructure in surgical ergonomics: a review of tasks, models, and measurement systems. Surg Innov 2007; 14(3): 153–67.

[24] Youssef Y, Lee G, Godinez C, Sutton E, Klein R V., George IM, et al. Laparoscopic cholecystectomy poses physical injury risk to surgeons: analysis of hand technique and standing position. Surg Endosc 2011; 25: 2168–74.

[25] Jack D, Boian R, Merians AS, Tremaine M, Burdea GC, Adamovich SV, Recce M, Poizner H. Virtual reality-enhanced stroke rehabilitation. IEEE Trans Neural Syst Rehabil Eng 2001; 9(3): 308–18.

[26] Stalfors J, Kling-Petersen T, Rydmark M, Westin T. Haptic palpation of head and neck cancer patients—implication for education and telemedicine. Stud Health Technol Inform 2001; 81: 471–4.

[27] Sánchez-Margallo FM, Sánchez-Margallo JA, Pagador JB, Moyano JL, Moreno J, Usón J. Ergonomic assessment of hand movements in laparoscopic surgery using the CyberGlove. In: Miller K, Nielsen PMF, editors. Comput. Biomech. Med., New York, NY: Springer; 2010, pp. 121–8.

[28] Hermens HJ, Freriks B, Merletti R, Stegeman D, Blok J, Rau G, et al. SENIAM 8: European recommendation for surface electromyography. Enschede: Roessingh Research and Development. 1999.

[29] Pérez-Duarte FJ, Sánchez-Margallo FM, Martín-Portugués I, Sánchez-Hurtado MA, Lucas-Hernández M, Sánchez-Margallo JA, et al. Ergonomic analysis of muscle activity in the forearm and back muscles during laparoscopic surgery. Surg Laparosc Endosc Percutan Tech 2013; 23: 203–7.

[30] Szeto GPY, Ho P, Ting CW, Poon JTC, Tsang RCC, Cheng SWK. A study of surgeons' postural muscle activity during open, laparoscopic, and endovascular surgery. Surg Endosc 2010; 24: 1712–21.

[31] Büchel D, Mårvik R, Hallabrin B, Matern U. Ergonomics of disposable handles for minimally invasive surgery. Surg Endosc 2010; 24: 992–1004.

[32] Fan Y, Kong G, Meng Y, Tan S, Wei K, Zhang Q, et al. Comparative assessment of surgeons' task performance and surgical ergonomics associated with conventional and modified flank positions: a simulation study. Surg Endosc 2014; 28: 3249–56.

[33] Wilson MR, Poolton JM, Malhotra N, Ngo K, Bright E, Masters RSW. Development and validation of a surgical workload measure: the surgery task load index (SURG-TLX). World J Surg 2011; 35: 1961–9.

[34] Abdelrahman AM, Bingener J, Yu D, Lowndes BR, Mohamed A, McConico AL, et al. Impact of single-incision laparoscopic cholecystectomy (SILC) versus conventional laparoscopic cholecystectomy (CLC) procedures on surgeon stress and workload: a randomized controlled trial. Surg Endosc 2016; 30: 1205–11.

[35] Hu JSL, Lu J, Tan WB, Lomanto D. Training improves laparoscopic tasks performance and decreases operator workload. Surg Endosc 2016; 30: 1742–6.

[36] Liang B, Qi L, Yang J, Cao Z, Zu X, Liu L, Wang L. Ergonomic status of laparoscopic urologic surgery: survey results from 241 urologic surgeons in china. PLoS One 2013; 8(7): e70423.

[37] Cass GK, Vyas S, Akande V. Prolonged laparoscopic surgery is associated with an increased risk of vertebral disc prolapse. J Obstet Gynaecol 2014; 34(1): 74–8.

[38] Franasiak J, Ko EM, Kidd J, Secord AA, Bell M, Boggess JF, Gehrig PA. Physical strain and urgent need for ergonomic training among gynecologic oncologists who perform minimally invasive surgery. Gynecol Oncol 2012; 126(3): 437–42.

[39] Sutton E, Irvin M, Zeigler C, Lee G, Park A. The ergonomics of women in surgery. Surg Endosc 2014; 28(4): 1051–5.

[40] Lucas-Hernández M, Pagador JB, Pérez-Duarte FJ, Castelló P, Sánchez-Margallo FM. Ergonomics problems due to the use and design of dissector and needle holder. Surg Laparosc Endosc Percutan Tech 2014; 24: e170–7.

[41] Filisetti C, Cho A, Riccipetitoni G, Saxena AK. Analysis of hand size and ergonomics of instruments in pediatric minimally invasive surgery. Surg Laparosc Endosc Percutan Tech 2015; 25(5): e159–62.

[42] Nieboer TE, Massa M, Weinans MJN, Vierhout ME, Kluivers KB, Stegeman DF. Does training of the nondominant upper extremity reduce the surgeon's muscular strain during laparoscopy?: Results from a randomized controlled trial. Surg Innov 2013; 20: 292–8.

[43] Haramis G, Rosales JC, Palacios JM, Okhunov Z, Mues AC, Lee D, et al. Prospective randomized evaluation of FOOT gel pads for operating room staff COMFORT during laparoscopic renal surgery. Urology 2010; 76: 1405–8.

[44] Yurko YY, Scerbo MW, Prabhu AS, Acker CE, Stefanidis D. Higher mental workload is associated with poorer laparoscopic performance as measured by the NASA-TLX tool. Simul Healthc 2010; 5(5): 267–71.

[45] Riggle JD, Miller EE, McCrory B, Meitl A, Lim E, Hallbeck MS, et al. Ergonomic comparison of laparoscopic hand instruments in a single site surgery simulator with novices. Minim Invasive Ther Allied Technol 2015; 24: 68–76.

[46] Bertolaccini L, Viti A, Terzi A. Ergon-trial: ergonomic evaluation of single-port access versus three-port access video-assisted thoracic surgery. Surg Endosc 2015; 29: 2934–40.

[47] Aubdoollah TH. Clinical outcomes and ergonomics analysis of three laparoscopic techniques for Hirschsprung's disease. World J Gastroenterol 2015; 21: 8903.

[48] Tsai Y-C, Lin VC-H, Chung S-D, Ho C-H, Jaw F-S, Tai H-C. Ergonomic and geometric tricks of laparoendoscopic single-site surgery (LESS) by using conventional laparoscopic instruments. Surg Endosc 2012; 26: 2671–7.

[49] Lee GI, Lee MR, Clanton T, Clanton T, Sutton E, Park AE, et al. Comparative assessment of physical and cognitive ergonomics associated with robotic and traditional laparoscopic surgeries. Surg Endosc 2014; 28: 456–65.

[50] Stefanidis D, Wang F, Korndorffer JR, Dunne JB, Scott DJ. Robotic assistance improves intracorporeal suturing performance and safety in the operating room while decreasing operator workload. Surg Endosc 2010; 24: 377–82.

[51] Moore LJ, Wilson MR, McGrath JS, Waine E, Masters RSW, Vine SJ. Surgeons' display reduced mental effort and workload while performing robotically assisted surgical tasks, when compared to conventional laparoscopy. Surg Endosc 2015; 29: 2553–60.

[52] Passerotti CC, Franco F, Bissoli JCC, Tiseo B, Oliveira CM, Buchalla CAO, et al. Comparison of the learning curves and frustration level in performing laparoscopic and robotic training skills by experts and novices. Int Urol Nephrol 2015; 47: 1075–84.

[53] Rousek JB, Brown-Clerk B, Lowndes BR, Balogh BJ, Hallbeck MS. Optimizing integration of electrosurgical hand controls within a laparoscopic surgical tool. Minim Invasive Ther Allied Technol 2012; 21: 222–33.

[54] Steinhilber B, Seibt R, Reiff F, Rieger MA, Kraemer B, Rothmund R. Effect of a laparoscopic instrument with rotatable handle piece on biomechanical stress during laparoscopic procedures. Surg Endosc 2016; 30: 78–88.

[55] Yu D, Lowndes B, Morrow M, Kaufman K, Bingener J, Hallbeck S. Impact of novel shift handle laparoscopic tool on wrist ergonomics and task performance. Surg Endosc 2015. [Epub ahead of print].

[56] Di Lorenzo N, Camperchioli I, Gaspari AL. Radius surgical system and conventional laparoscopic instruments in abdominal surgery: application, learning curve and ergonomy. Surg Oncol 2007;16(Suppl 1): S69–72.

[57] Hirano Y, Inaki N, Ishikawa N, Watanabe G. Laparoscopic treatment for esophageal achalasia and gastro-esophago-reflex disease using radius surgical system. Indian J Surg 2013; 75: 160–2.

[58] Gözen AS, Tokas T, Tschada A, Jalal A, Klein J, Rassweiler J. Direct comparison of the different conventional laparoscopic positions with the ethos surgical platform in a laparoscopic pelvic surgery simulation setting. J Endourol 2015; 29: 95–9.

[59] Steinhilber B, Hoffmann S, Karlovic K, Pfeffer S, Maier T, Hallasheh O, et al. Development of an arm support system to improve ergonomics in laparoscopic surgery: study design and provisional results. Surg Endosc 2015; 29: 2851–8.

[60] Xiao D, Jakimowicz JJ, Albayrak A, Buzink SN, Botden SMBI, Goossens RHM. Face, content, and construct validity of a novel portable ergonomic simulator for basic laparoscopic skills. J Surg Educ 2014; 71: 65–72.

Chapter 6

Diagnostic Laparoscopy for Abdominal Tuberculosis: A Promising Tool for Diagnosis

Arshad M. Malik

Additional information is available at the end of the chapter

http://dx.doi.org/10.5772/64611

Abstract

Introduction: Abdominal tuberculosis has plagued the mankind over several decades and is a major reason of morbidity and mortality even today in the developing world. It's a difficult problem to diagnose as most patients present with vague and nonspecific symptomatology. This study was performed with a view to find out an efficient and practical tool for diagnosing this problem.

Methods: This analytical descriptive study including 283 patients of abdominal tuberculosis is a continuation of an earlier study by the author in the same context. The study was conducted to highlight the usefulness of diagnostic laparoscopy in patients with vague abdominal symptoms, posing difficulty in establishing a conclusive diagnosis. The study extended over a nine-year period in a teaching hospital as well as some private hospitals. The data was collected and statistically analyzed on SPSS version 22.

Results: We had a total of 266 patients with unsettled diagnosis having vague abdominal symptoms. Out of the total study subjects, 214 (80.45%) were finally conclusively diagnosed to have abdominal tuberculosis on diagnostic laparoscopy. Abdominal pain is the most frequent symptom which makes the patients seek medical advice coupled with changing bowel habits, loss of weight and generalized weakness. Laparoscopy revealed various tuberculous lesions which were biopsied and diagnosed.

Conclusion: Diagnostic laparoscopy is a potential answer for the diagnostic dilemma posed by abdominal tuberculosis. Its efficacy and reliability need further studies in future.

Keywords: abdominal tuberculosis, diagnostic dilemma, morbidity, cost-effectiveness

1. Background

Abdominal tuberculosis remains one of the commonest and most difficult diseases globally as far as the diagnosis is concerned [1–5]. It is also one of the common extra-pulmonary sites for tuberculous lesions. The disease may affect any part of the gut and may produce a chronic illness with vague abdominal symptoms or else may present in an acute obstructive form. The gravity of this problem is further increased by the vague and totally non-specific symptomatology [6–7]. The presentation of abdominal tuberculosis always mimics many other conditions like inflammatory bowel diseases and other similar conditions [8–10]. This state of confusion usually leads to an undue delay in diagnosis and treatment plan and thus further increases the overall morbidity. A large number of these patients present with acute abdomen and are diagnosed on exploratory laparotomy only. This actually has been a practice in our setup where a large number of patients undergo unnecessary laparotomies. These laparotomies could be easily avoided had there been an efficient and reliable method to diagnose abdominal tuberculosis. This actually led to the consideration of diagnostic laparoscopy in all patients with suspected abdominal tuberculosis to find out tuberculous lesions and to take biopsy of any such foci. This proved to be a breakthrough with a very encouraging result [11–13]. The study focused on the possible role of laparoscopy to establish the histopathological diagnosis of tuberculosis in patients having a high degree of suspicion but we found it difficult to establish a concrete diagnosis. Early diagnosis and starting anti-tuberculous diagnosis and an early resort to the anti-tuberculous treatment can coma after morbidity can facilitate an early recovery and an early return to work. This has a lot of benefits to the patient, the community and a major cut short on the health facility.

1.2. Pathology and pathogenesis

Tuberculosis is a common problem in developing countries like Pakistan, India, Bangladesh, etc. In the early 1990s, it was considered a lethal disease as there were no medications effective against the tubercle bacillus. With the advent of anti-tuberculous drugs, the disease is no more a problem as it used to be in the past. The disease represents one of the most dreaded forms of extra-pulmonary disease and can affect virtually all parts of the GIT including intestines and various abdominal viscera.

The portal of entry of mycobacterium into the GIT is through ingestion of the infected sputum, via blood, or there may be a direct spread from infected contiguous organs like fallopian tubes, etc. [14]. The abdominal tuberculosis is divided into the following categories based on the gross appearance and involvement of the target tissue.

A. Intestinal tuberculosis

B. Glandular tuberculosis

C. Peritoneal tuberculosis

D. Solid organs

http://dx.doi.org/10.5772/64611

Rathi et al. [15] claim that abdominal tuberculosis constitutes 11% of the extra-pulmonary sites and the commonest area affected is the ileocecal region. The intestinal tuberculosis usually has three gross pathological forms as under

a. Hypertrophied

b. Ulcerative

c. Stricturous

The ileocecal tuberculosis is always a hypertrophied lesion which may present with acute intestinal obstruction. The ulcerative lesion is in the form of mucosal ulcers which usually present with diarrhoea and other abdominal symptoms. There is a recent claim that the extra-pulmonary manifestations of tuberculosis are observed with increasing frequency in Immuno-suppressed patients and more so with HIV patients as an accompaniment of the chronic illness [16]. An early diagnosis is the key to a curable non-operative treatment as a vast majority of these patients can be treated by anti-tuberculous drugs and thus can be saved from an undue laparotomy. In order to achieve this goal, the first and the foremost thing is to have a high index of suspicion about this entity [17] coupled with expertise in the laparoscopic technique.

2. Methods

This analytical descriptive study was conducted in a teaching hospital as well as some private hospitals. The study subjects attended the outpatient department with acute or chronic presentations. Patients having a totally confusing symptomatology and vague symptoms where a firm conclusive diagnosis could not be established were included in the study and were informed about the purpose of the study and the possible outcome. Having learnt the objectives of the study, only those who gave their consent were enrolled and admitted in the hospital. Patients who were already diagnosed as ileocecal tuberculosis or were on anti-tuberculous treatment were excluded. Upon arrival, the initial management was totally determined by the mode of presentation. Patients with acute presentation were resuscitated with I/V fluids and decompressed by nasogastric suction to stabilize for intervention. The patients who presented with vague abdominal symptoms were thoroughly examined and were given conservative treatment to correct body fluids and electrolytes and to relieve pain.

After having done the initial resuscitation and management, investigations were sent including blood complete picture, chest x-ray, abdominal x-rays, ultrasound examination and CT scan in some patients. Failing to achieve a conclusive clue on abdominal examination and investigations, a diagnostic laparoscopy was planned, keeping in view a very high incidence of the tuberculosis in our part of the world. The various variables studied included demographics, clinical presentations, common laboratory results and outcomes of diagnostic laparoscopy.

3. Results

Of the total study subjects, 266 patients were chosen for diagnostic laparoscopy based on the fact that their findings and symptomatology were so vague that a conclusion could not be drawn from the clinical examination and the usual laboratory workup. The demographics included 186 (70%) males and 80 (30%) females with a mean age of 36.59, range of 48 (17–65) and a standard deviation of 10.875. The main symptoms and the mode of presentation of the patients are shown in **Table 1**. The minimum duration of the symptoms was found to be eight days (3%), while the maximum duration of symptoms was found to be > 1 month (43%). A vast majority (81%) of the patients were found to have haemoglobin < 10 G%. Ultrasound examination was not a very helpful tool as depicted in **Table 2**. The Mantoux test was positive only in eight (3%) patients while 97% had a negative Mantoux. Erythrocyte sedimentation rate (ESR) was raised in a high number of patients (97%). Generalised tenderness of abdomen and weakness was present in 88% of the study population, while the remaining patients had insignificant examination findings. Chest x-ray was absolutely normal in 250 (94%) of the total study subjects. The various laparoscopic findings are shown in **Table 3**. One hundred and seventy-eight (67%) patients had a positive history of taking off and on anti-tuberculous medication prescribed by the local general practitioners. Most of the patients, referred from far flung areas, referred from remote far flung areas had positive laparoscopic findings compared to the urban population ($p < 0.001$). Of the total population, we were able to confirm histopathological diagnosis in 259 patients having different forms of abdominal tuberculosis. The various tuberculous findings on laparoscopy are found in **Figures 1–3**. Stricturous pathology and obstructive ileocecal tuberculosis needed operative intervention in 23 (9%) patients while remaining patients received a full course of anti-tuberculous drugs and showed full recovery. A follow-up of these patients was carried for a period of three years.

	Main symptoms			
	Sub-acute intestinal obstruction	**Vague abdominal pain and loss of weight**	**Chronic off-and on-obstruction**	**Total**
Mode of presentation				
Acute	0	0	12	12
Chronic	2	180	0	182
Acute-on-chronic	66	0	6	72
Total	68	180	18	266

Table 1. Mode of presentations and main symptoms.

	Frequency	**Percentage**	**Total**
Inconclusive	150	56	
Diagnosed tuberculosis	34	12.78	266
Gave suspicion of tuberculosis	82	30	

Table 2. Ultrasound abdomen results.

Finding	Frequency	Percentage
No abnormality detected	52	19
Miliary tuberculosis found	104	39
Mesenteric lymphadenopathy detected	90	34
Intestinal strictures found	20	7.5

Table 3. Various laparoscopic findings.

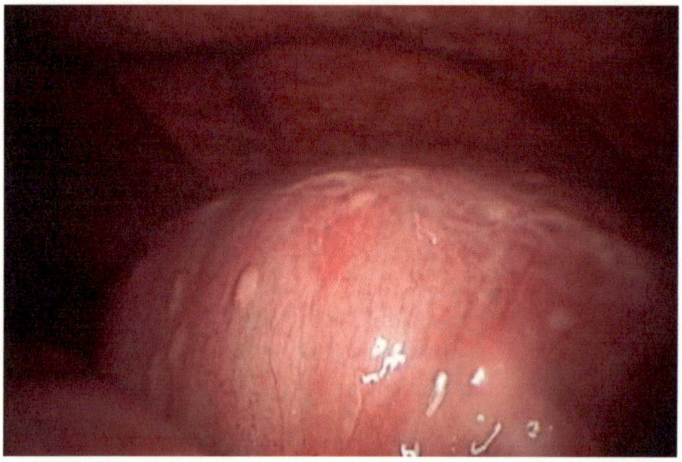

Figure 1. Miliary tubercles on the intestinal wall and abdominal wall.

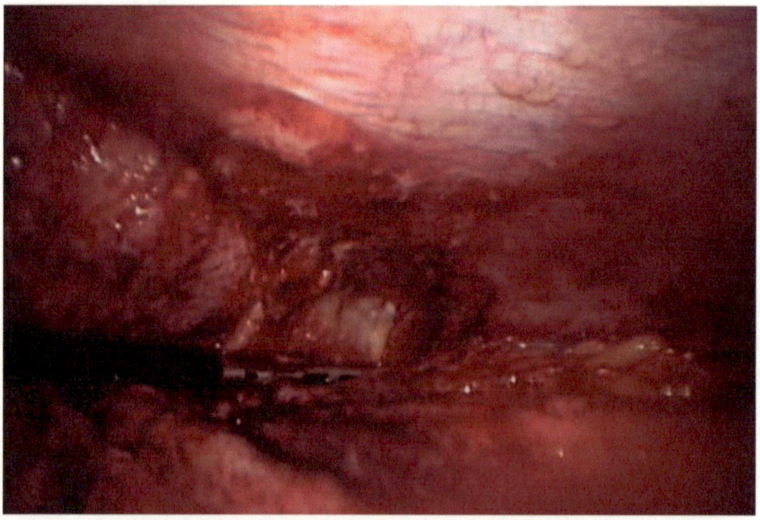

Figure 2. Plastic adhesions.

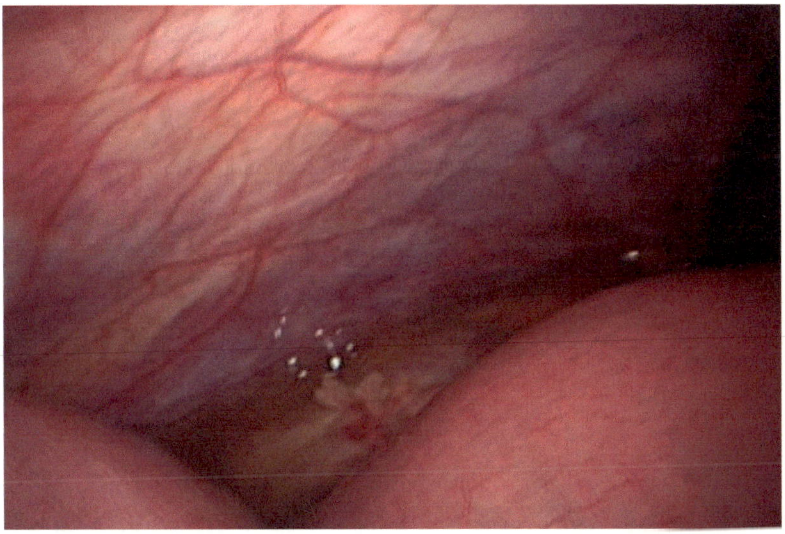

Figure 3. Ascitic fluid.

3.1. Difficulties and limitations

Although apparently an excellent diagnostic tool for the diagnosis of abdominal tuberculosis, at times we faced a lot of problems especially when there are severe plastic adhesions and more so when you find an abdominal cocoon. It is usually very difficult to introduce the first trocar in such situations.

4. Discussion

Abdominal tuberculosis remains a difficult major health issue all over the world. It is highly challenging and a dreaded problem for surgeons working in far-flung remote areas with limited resources and facilities. It is a diagnostic challenge for surgeons globally but more so in the third-world countries where the disease is rife and remains unnoticed till it turns into a serious emergency. The abdominal tuberculosis is known for its varied and confusing symptomatology whereby it mimics closely with various other similar diseases like inflammatory bowel diseases [18–19]. The unusual presentation and confusion in diagnosis usually lead to unnecessary and avoidable laparotomies, which is most of the time performed as a last resort to reach to a conclusive diagnosis. Contrary to the earlier reports, the developing countries are showing a fearful increase in the incidence of abdominal tuberculosis, as reported in recent studies [20–22]. The increase in the prevalence of abdominal tuberculosis in the developing countries is attributed to a rising incidence of HIV-positive population linking it to immunosuppression [12, 19].The age incidence of our study population coincides with other similar reports [20]. The male dominance is very clear in our studies as reported by other similar studies [18]. The varied presentation is the hallmark of abdominal tuberculosis, and as

shown in our results, it is also consistent with and reported by other similar reports [23–24]. Our study highlights the fact that there is a very alarmingly high incidence of this disease in the poor, underprivileged rural population of Sind province of Pakistan. It is highly recommended to have a high level of suspicion to reach a conclusive diagnosis whenever a patient presents with vague abdominal symptoms [25]. There is hardly any absolutely reliable diagnostic test that can give a 100% confirmed diagnosis of abdominal tuberculosis. This simply is the reason for an unnecessary and life-threatening delay in the diagnosis of this disease [8, 26]. The diagnostic laparoscopy and biopsy of the tuberculous lesions are not a recent advancement but are rather known for over 30 years now [27]. It however has not been practiced widely and as commonly as it should have been. Even today, this diagnostic tool has not attracted the desired level of attention and usually is considered a last resort rather than the first in difficult diagnostic situations. In the current study, we gave it a place of primary investigation tool along with other diagnostic tests and we found it extremely encouraging as the yield of diagnosis is over 80%, in line with other similar studies [28–29]. Diagnostic laparoscopy prompts the diagnosis and can reduce the delay which can increase the morbidity and can lead to unnecessary laparotomies while improving the outcome [30–31]. Despite all the benefits, some limitations like a deceiving view leading to mis-diagnosis regardless of the experience of surgeon are mentioned by few studies [32–35].

5. Conclusion

The diagnostic laparoscopy in suspected cases of abdominal tuberculosis is an efficient and rewarding method of diagnosis. A regular use of this diagnostic modality can improve the overall outlook of this common disease in the developing world.

Author details

Arshad M. Malik

Address all correspondence to: arshadhamzapk@yahoo.com

College of Medicine, Qassim University, Saudi Arabia

References

[1] Aston NO. Abdominal tuberculosis. World J Surg 1997; 21(5):492–9.

[2] Rai S, Thomas WM. Diagnosis of abdominal tuberculosis: The importance of laparoscopy. J R Soc Med 2003; 96:586–8.

[3] Bouma BJ, Tytgat KMAJ, Shipper HG, Kager PA. Be aware of abdominal tuberculosis. Neth J Med 1997; 51:119–22.

[4] Shakil AO, Korula J, Kanel GC, Murray NGB, Reynolds TB. Diagnostic features of tuberculous peritonitis in the absence and presence of chronic liver disease: A case control study. Am J Med 1996; 100:179–85.

[5] Sinkala E, Gray S, Zulu I, Mudenda V, Zimba L, Vermund SH, Droniewski F, Kelly P. Clinical and ultrasonological features of abdominal tuberculosis in HIV positive adults in Zambia. BMC Infect Dis 2009; 9:44.

[6] Uygur-Bayramicli O, Dabak G, Babak R. A clinical dilemma: Abdominal tuberculosis. World J Gastroenterol 2003; 9(5):1098–101.

[7] Krishnan P, Vayoth SO, Dhar P et al. Laparoscopy in suspected abdominal tuberculosis is useful as an early diagnostic method. ANZ J Surg 2008; 78(11):987–9.

[8] Akcam M, Artan R, Yilmaz A, Cig H, Aksoy NH. Abdominal tuberculosis in adolescents. Difficulties in diagnosis. Saudi Med J 2005; 26(1):122–6.

[9] Ramesh J, Banait GS, Ormerod LP. Abdominal tuberculosis in a district general hospital: A retrospective review of 86 cases. Q J Med 2008; 101:189–95.

[10] Jaydyar H, Mindelzun RE, Olcott EW, Levitt DB. Still a great mimicker: Abdominal tuberculosis. Am J Radiol 1997; 168:1455–60.

[11] Salky BA, Edye MB. The role of laparoscopy in the diagnosis and treatment of abdominal of abdominal pain syndromes. Surg Endosc 1998; 7(12):911–4.

[12] McLaughin S, Jones T, Pitcher M, Evans P. Laparoscopic diagnosis of abdominal tuberculosis. ANZ J Surg 2008; 68(8):599–601.

[13] Sharma MP, Bhatia V. Abdominal tuberculosis. Indian J Med Res. 2004; 120(4):305–15.

[14] Rathi P, Gambhire P. Abdominal tuberculosis. J Assoc Physicians India. 2016; 64(2):38–47.

[15] Kienzl-Palma D, Prosch H. Extrathoracic manifestations of tuberculosis. Radiologe. 2016; 56(10):885–9.

[16] Debi U, Ravisankar V, Prasad KK, Sinha SK, Sharma AK. Abdominal tuberculosis of the gastrointestinal tract: Revisited. World J Gastroenterol. 2014; 20(40):14831–40. doi:10.3748/wjg.v20.i40.14831.

[17] Sinan T, Sheikh M, Ramadan S, Sahwney S, Behbehani A. CT features in abdominal tuberculosis: 20 years experience. BMC Med Imag 2002; 2(1):3.

[18] Jadvar H, Mindelzun RE, Olcott EW, Levitt DB. Still the great mimicker: Abdominal tuberculosis. Am J Roentgenol 1997; 168:1455–60.

[19] Navaneethan U, Cherian JV, Prabhu R, Venkataraman J. Distinguishing tuberculosis and Crohn's disease in developing countries: How certain can you be of the diagnosis? Saudi J Gastroenterol 2009; 15(2):142–4.

[20] Kapoor V. Abdominal tuberculosis. Medicine 2009; 35(5):257–60.

[21] Kishore PV, Palaian S, chandersekhar TS. Diagnosing tuberculosis. A retrospective study from Nepal. Internet J Gastroenterol 2008; 6(2):1–6

[22] Al Karawi MA, Mohammed AE, Yasawy MI, Graham DY, Shariq S, Ahmed AM et al. Protean manifestations of gastrointestinal tuberculosis; report on 130 patients. J Clin Gastroenterol 1995; 20(3):225–32.

[23] Tan KK, Chen K, Sim R. The spectrum of abdominal tuberculosis in a developed country: A single institutions experience over 7 years. J Gatroentrointest Surg 2009; 13(1):142–7.

[24] Vyravanathan S, Jeyarajah R. Tuberculous peritonitis: A review of thirty-five cases. Post Grad Med J 1980; 56(659):649–51.

[25] Uzunkoy A, Harma M, Harma M. Diagnosis of abdominal tuberculosis: Experience from 11 cases and review of the literature. World J Gasteroenterol 2004; 10(24):3647–9.

[26] Al Muneef M, Memish Z, Al Mahmoud S, Al Sadoon S, Bannatyne R, Khan Y. Tuberculosis in the belly: A review of forty six cases involving the gastrointestinal tract and peritoneum. Scand J Gastroenterol 2001; 36(5):528–32.

[27] Tarcoveanu E, Flip V, Moldovanu R, Dimofte G, Lupascu C, Vlad N et al. Abdominal tuberculosis- a surgical reality. Chirurgia (Bucur) 2007; 102(3):303–8.

[28] Machado N, Grant CS, Scrimgeour E. Abdominal tuberculosis—experience of a university hospital in Oman. Acta Trop 2001; 80(2):187–90.

[29] Trujillo NP. Peritoneoscopy and guided biopsy in the diagnosis of intra abdominal diseases. Gastroentrology 1976; 71:1083–5.

[30] Singh-Ranger D. Diagnosis of abdominal tuberculosis. J R Soc Med 2004; 97:154–7.

[31] Udwadia TE. Diagnostic laparoscopy. Surg Endosc 2004; 18(1):6–10.

[32] Al-Akeely MH. Impact of elective diagnostic laparoscopy in chronic abdominal disorders. Saudi J Gastroentrol 2006; 12(1):27–30.

[33] Cached J, Mekki M, Mansour A, Ben Brahim M, Maazoun K, Hidouri S et al. Contribution of laparoscopy in abdominal tuberculosis diagnosis: Retrospective study of about 11 cases. Pediatr Surg Int 2010; 26(4):413–8.

[34] Tarcoveanu E, Dimofte G, Bradea C, Lupascu C, Moldovanu R, Vasilescu A. Peritoneal tuberculosis in laparoscopic era. Acta Chir Belg 2009; 109(1):65–70.

[35] Meshikhes AW. Pitfalls of diagnostic laparoscopy in abdominal tuberculosis. Surg Endosc 2010; 24(4):908–10.